AF784771

Exploring the Current Landscape of Consumer Genomics

PROCEEDINGS OF A WORKSHOP

Meredith Hackmann, Siobhan Addie, Joe Alper, and Sarah H. Beachy,
Rapporteurs

Roundtable on Genomics and Precision Health

Board on Health Sciences Policy

Health and Medicine Division

The National Academies of
SCIENCES · ENGINEERING · MEDICINE

THE NATIONAL ACADEMIES PRESS
Washington, DC
www.nap.edu

THE NATIONAL ACADEMIES PRESS 500 Fifth Street, NW Washington, DC 20001

This project was supported by contracts between the National Academy of Sciences and 23andMe; Air Force Medical Service (Contract No. FA8052-17-P-0007); American Academy of Nursing; American College of Medical Genetics and Genomics; American Medical Association; Association for Molecular Pathology; Biogen; Blue Cross and Blue Shield Association; College of American Pathologists; Color Genomics; Department of Veterans Affairs (Contract No. VA240-14-C-0037); Eisai Inc.; Geisinger; Genosity; Health Resources and Services Administration (Contract No. HHSH250201500001I/HHSH25034003T/0003); Helix; Illumina, Inc.; The Jackson Laboratory; Janssen Research & Development, LLC; Merck & Co., Inc. (Contract No. CMO-180815-002787); Myriad Women's Health; National Institutes of Health (Contract No. HHSN263201800029I/Order No. HHSN26300010): All of Us Research Program, National Cancer Institute, National Human Genome Research Institute, National Institute of Mental Health, National Institute of Nursing Research, National Institute on Aging, Office of Disease Prevention; National Society of Genetic Counselors; Pfizer Inc.; Regeneron; The University of Vermont Health Network Medical Group; and Vibrent Health. Any opinions, findings, conclusions, or recommendations expressed in this publication do not necessarily reflect the views of any organization or agency that provided support for the project.

International Standard Book Number-13: 978-0-309-67303-7
International Standard Book Number-10: 0-309-67303-8
Digital Object Identifier: https://doi.org/10.17226/25713

Additional copies of this publication are available from the National Academies Press, 500 Fifth Street, NW, Keck 360, Washington, DC 20001; (800) 624-6242 or (202) 334-3313; http://www.nap.edu.

Printed in the United States of America

Suggested citation: National Academies of Sciences, Engineering, and Medicine. 2020. *Exploring the current landscape of consumer genomics: Proceedings of a workshop*. Washington, DC: The National Academies Press. https://doi.org/10.17226/25713.

The National Academies of
SCIENCES • ENGINEERING • MEDICINE

The **National Academy of Sciences** was established in 1863 by an Act of Congress, signed by President Lincoln, as a private, nongovernmental institution to advise the nation on issues related to science and technology. Members are elected by their peers for outstanding contributions to research. Dr. Marcia McNutt is president.

The **National Academy of Engineering** was established in 1964 under the charter of the National Academy of Sciences to bring the practices of engineering to advising the nation. Members are elected by their peers for extraordinary contributions to engineering. Dr. John L. Anderson is president.

The **National Academy of Medicine** (formerly the Institute of Medicine) was established in 1970 under the charter of the National Academy of Sciences to advise the nation on medical and health issues. Members are elected by their peers for distinguished contributions to medicine and health. Dr. Victor J. Dzau is president.

The three Academies work together as the **National Academies of Sciences, Engineering, and Medicine** to provide independent, objective analysis and advice to the nation and conduct other activities to solve complex problems and inform public policy decisions. The National Academies also encourage education and research, recognize outstanding contributions to knowledge, and increase public understanding in matters of science, engineering, and medicine.

Learn more about the National Academies of Sciences, Engineering, and Medicine at **www.nationalacademies.org.**

The National Academies of

SCIENCES · ENGINEERING · MEDICINE

Consensus Study Reports published by the National Academies of Sciences, Engineering, and Medicine document the evidence-based consensus on the study's statement of task by an authoring committee of experts. Reports typically include findings, conclusions, and recommendations based on information gathered by the committee and the committee's deliberations. Each report has been subjected to a rigorous and independent peer-review process and it represents the position of the National Academies on the statement of task.

Proceedings published by the National Academies of Sciences, Engineering, and Medicine chronicle the presentations and discussions at a workshop, symposium, or other event convened by the National Academies. The statements and opinions contained in proceedings are those of the participants and are not endorsed by other participants, the planning committee, or the National Academies.

For information about other products and activities of the National Academies, please visit www.nationalacademies.org/about/whatwedo.

PLANNING COMMITTEE ON EXPLORING THE CURRENT LANDSCAPE OF CONSUMER GENOMICS[1]

W. GREGORY FEERO (*Co-Chair*), Associate Editor and Representative of *JAMA*; Professor, Department of Community and Family Medicine, Geisel School of Medicine; Faculty, Maine Dartmouth Family Medicine Residency Program, Fairfield, ME
CATHY WICKLUND (*Co-Chair*), Past President, National Society of Genetic Counselors; Director, Graduate Program in Genetic Counseling; Associate Professor, Feinberg School of Medicine, Center for Genetic Medicine, Northwestern University, Evanston, IL
BRUCE BLUMBERG, Professor of Clinical Science and Planning Co-Lead of Faculty Development, Kaiser Permanente School of Medicine
NATASHA BONHOMME, Chief Strategy Officer, Genetic Alliance
AARON GOLDENBERG, Associate Professor and Research Director, Department of Bioethics and Medical Humanities, Case Western Reserve University School of Medicine
GEORGE MENSAH, Director, Center for Translation Research and Implementation Science, National Heart, Lung, and Blood Institute, National Institutes of Health
VICTORIA PRATT, Representative of the Association for Molecular Pathology; Director, Pharmacogenomics and Molecular Genetics Laboratories, Department of Medical and Molecular Genetics, School of Medicine, Indiana University, Indianapolis, IN
DONNA ROSCOE, Supervisory Biologist, Center for Devices and Radiological Health, Food and Drug Administration
JACQUELYN TAYLOR, Professor of Nursing, Medicine, and Population Health; Vernice Ferguson Endowed Chair in Health Equity; Director, Meyers Biological Laboratory, New York University College of Nursing and School of Medicine
JOYCE TUNG, Vice President, Research, 23andMe

Roundtable on Genomics and Precision Health Staff

SARAH H. BEACHY, Senior Program Officer and Roundtable Director
SIOBHAN ADDIE, Program Officer

---

[1]The National Academies of Sciences, Engineering, and Medicine's planning committees are solely responsible for organizing the workshop, identifying topics, and choosing speakers. The responsibility for the published proceedings of a workshop rests with the workshop rapporteurs and the institution.

MEREDITH HACKMANN, Associate Program Officer
MICHAEL BERRIOS, Senior Program Assistant

Board on Health Sciences Policy Staff

BRIDGET BOREL, Administrative Assistant (*from October 2019*)
MARIAM SHELTON, Program Coordinator (*until October 2019*)
ANDREW M. POPE, Senior Board Director

ROUNDTABLE ON GENOMICS AND PRECISION HEALTH[1]

GEOFFREY GINSBURG (*Co-Chair*), Director, Center for Applied Genomics and Precision Medicine; Director, MEDx; Professor of Medicine and Pathology, Duke University School of Medicine; Professor of Biomedical Engineering, Duke Pratt School of Engineering, Professor in School of Nursing, Duke University, Durham, NC

MICHELLE PENNY (*Co-Chair*), Senior Director and Head of the Translational Genome Sciences Group, Biogen, Boston, MA

NAOMI ARONSON, Executive Director, Technology Evaluation Center, Blue Cross and Blue Shield Association, Chicago, IL

ARIS BARAS, Senior Vice President, Regeneron Pharmaceuticals; General Manager, Regeneron Genetics Center, Tarrytown, NY

KARINA BIENFAIT, Principal Scientist, Clinical Pharmacogenomics and Operations, and Head, Global Genomics Policy, Process, and Compliance, Merck and Co., Inc., Kenilworth, NJ

VENCE BONHAM, Senior Advisor to the National Human Genome Research Institute Director on Genomics and Health Disparities, National Human Genome Research Institute, National Institutes of Health, Bethesda, MD

ANN CASHION (*until September 2019*), Scientific Director, and Acting Director, National Institute of Nursing Research, National Institutes of Health, Bethesda, MD

ROBERT B. DARNELL, Heilbrunn Cancer Professor and Senior Physician, Head, Laboratory of Molecular Neuro-Oncology, The Rockefeller University; Investigator, Howard Hughes Medical Institute; Founding Director and Chief Executive Officer Emeritus, New York Genome Center, New York, NY

STEPHANIE DEVANEY (*from September 2019*), Chief Operating Officer, All of Us Research Program, National Institutes of Health, Bethesda, MD

KATHERINE DONIGAN, Deputy Director (acting), Personalized Medicine and Molecular Genetics, Center for Devices and Radiological Health, Office of In Vitro Diagnostics and Radiological Health, Food and Drug Administration, Silver Spring, MD

[1]The National Academies of Sciences, Engineering, and Medicine's forums and roundtables do not issue, review, or approve individual documents. The responsibility for the published proceedings of a workshop rests with the workshop rapporteurs and the institution.

W. GREGORY FEERO, Associate Editor and Representative of *JAMA*; Professor, Department of Community and Family Medicine, Geisel School of Medicine; Faculty, Maine Dartmouth Family Medicine Residency Program, Fairfield, ME

JESSICA GILL (*from October 2019*), Lasker Clinical Research Scholar, Tissue Injury Branch, Division of Intramural Research, National Institute of Nursing Research, National Institutes of Health, Bethesda, MD

MARC GRODMAN, Co-Founder and Chief Executive Officer, Genosity; Assistant Professor of Clinical Medicine, Columbia University, New York, NY

JILL M. HAGENKORD (*until September 2019*), Chief Medical Officer, Color Genomics, Mountain View, CA

EMILY HARRIS (*until December 2019*), Deputy Associate Director, Epidemiology and Genetics Research Program, Division of Cancer Control and Population Sciences, National Cancer Institute, Rockville, MD

RICHARD J. HODES, Director, National Institute on Aging, National Institutes of Health, Bethesda, MD

PRADUMAN JAIN, Chief Executive Officer, Vibrent Health, Fairfax, VA

SEKAR KATHIRESAN, Director, Center for Genomic Medicine, Massachusetts General Hospital, Boston, MA

MUIN KHOURY, Director, National Office of Public Health Genomics, Centers for Disease Control and Prevention, Atlanta, GA

DAVID LEDBETTER (*from January 2020*), Executive Vice President and Chief Scientific Officer, Geisinger, Danville, PA

CHARLES LEE (*from August 2019*), Scientific Director and Professor, The Jackson Laboratory for Genomic Medicine, Farmington, CT

THOMAS LEHNER, Director, Office of Genomics Research Coordination, National Institute of Mental Health, National Instistutes of Health, Bethesda, MD

DEBRA LEONARD (*from January 2020*), Representative of the College of American Pathologists; Chair, Pathology and Laboratory Medicine; Pathologist, Professor, and Chair, Department of Pathology, The University of Vermont Medical Center, Burlington, VT

PATRICK LOERCH, Vice President, Global Head Data Sciences & Prevention Biomarkers, World Without Disease Accelerator, Johnson & Johnson, Boston, MA

JAMES LU, Co-Founder and Chief Scientific Officer, Helix, San Mateo, CA

SEAN McCONNELL, Senior Policy Analyst, Genomics, American Medical Association, Chicago, IL

MONA MILLER (*from October 2019*), Executive Director, American Society of Human Genetics, Bethesda, MD

JENNIFER MOSER, Health Science Specialist, Genomic Medicine Program, Office of Research and Development, Department of Veterans Affairs, Washington, DC

ANNA PETTERSSON, Senior Director, Science Policy and Advocacy, Pfizer Inc., New York, NY

VICTORIA M. PRATT, Representative of the Association for Molecular Pathology; Director, Pharmacogenomics and Molecular Genetics Laboratories, Department of Medical and Molecular Genetics, School of Medicine, Indiana University, Indianapolis, IN

NADEEM SARWAR, President, Andover Product Creation Innovation System, Eisai Inc., Cambridge, MA

SHERI SCHULLY (*until August 2019*), Senior Advisor for Disease Prevention, Office of Disease Prevention, National Institutes of Health, Bethesda, MD

JOAN A. SCOTT, Director, Division of Services for Children with Special Health Needs, Maternal and Child Health Bureau, Health Resources and Services Administration, Rockville, MD

SAM SHEKAR (*until June 2019*), Chief Medical Officer, Health Information Technology Program, Northrop Grumman Information Systems, McLean, VA

NONNIEKAYE SHELBURNE (*from January 2020*), Program Director, Clinical and Translational Epidemiology Branch, Epidemiology and Genomics Research Program, National Cancer Institute, National Institutes of Health, Bethesda, MD

NIKOLETTA SIDIROPOULOS, Associate Professor, Department of Pathology and Laboratory Medicine; Director of Molecular Pathology, The University of Vermont Medical Center and The University of Vermont Health Network Medical Group, Burlington, VT

KATHERINE JOHANSEN TABER, Senior Director, Clinical Development, Myriad Women's Health, South San Francisco, CA

RYAN TAFT, Vice President, Scientific Research, Illumina, Inc., San Diego, CA

JACQUELYN TAYLOR, Professor of Nursing, Medicine, and Population Health; Vernice Ferguson Endowed Chair in Health Equity; Director, Meyers Biological Laboratory, New York University College of Nursing and School of Medicine, Brooklyn, NY

SHARON TERRY, Chief Executive Officer, Genetic Alliance, Washington, DC

JOYCE TUNG, Vice President, Research, 23andMe, Mountain View, CA

JAMESON VOSS, Chief, Air Force Medical Service Precision Medicine, Air Force Medical Support Agency, Falls Church, VA

Reviewers

This Proceedings of a Workshop was reviewed in draft form by individuals chosen for their diverse perspectives and technical expertise. The purpose of this independent review is to provide candid and critical comments that will assist the National Academies of Sciences, Engineering, and Medicine in making each published proceedings as sound as possible and to ensure that it meets the institutional standards for quality, objectivity, evidence, and responsiveness to the charge. The review comments and draft manuscript remain confidential to protect the integrity of the process.

We thank the following individuals for their review of this proceedings:

LIDA BENINSON, National Academies of Sciences, Engineering, and Medicine
KAREN WECK, University of North Carolina at Chapel Hill

Although the reviewers listed above provided many constructive comments and suggestions, they were not asked to endorse the content of the proceedings nor did they see the final draft before its release. The review of this proceedings was overseen by **BRUCE CALONGE,** The Colorado Trust. He was responsible for making certain that an independent examination of this proceedings was carried out in accordance with standards of the National Academies and that all review comments were carefully considered. Responsibility for the final content rests entirely with the rapporteurs and the National Academies.

Acknowledgments

The support of the Roundtable on Genomics and Precision Health was crucial to the planning and conduct of this workshop on Exploring the Current Landscape of Consumer Genomics. Federal sponsors for the workshop were the Air Force Medical Service; Department of Veterans Affairs; Health Resources and Services Administration; National Institutes of Health: All of Us Research Program, National Cancer Institute, National Human Genome Research Institute, National Institute of Mental Health, National Institute of Nursing Research, National Institute on Aging, and Office of Disease Prevention. Nonfederal sponsorship was provided by 23andMe; American Academy of Nursing; American College of Medical Genetics and Genomics; American Medical Association; Association for Molecular Pathology; Biogen; Blue Cross and Blue Shield Association; College of American Pathologists; Color Genomics; Eisai Inc.; Geisinger; Genosity; Helix; Illumina, Inc.; The Jackson Laboratory; Janssen Research & Development, LLC; Merck & Co., Inc.; Myriad Women's Health; National Society of Genetic Counselors; Pfizer Inc.; Regeneron; The University of Vermont Health Network Medical Group; and Vibrent Health.

The Roundtable on Genomics and Precision Health wishes to express gratitude to the members of the planning committee for their work in developing an excellent workshop agenda and to the expert speakers who explored the current state of consumer genomics and integration into the health care system. The project director would like to thank the project staff who worked diligently to develop both the workshop and the resulting proceedings.

Contents

Boxes, Figures, and Table

BOXES

FIGURES

TABLE

Acronyms and Abbreviations

ACA	Patient Protection and Affordable Care Act
ACLA	American Clinical Laboratory Association
ADA	Americans with Disabilities Act
AMP	Association for Molecular Pathology
CLIA	Clinical Laboratory Improvement Amendments
CMS	Centers for Medicare & Medicaid Services
DTC	direct-to-consumer
FBI	Federal Bureau of Investigation
FDA	Food and Drug Administration
FTC	Federal Trade Commission
GINA	Genetic Information Nondiscrimination Act
HIPAA	Health Insurance Portability and Accountability Act
LDT	laboratory-developed test
NHGRI	National Human Genome Research Institute
PGen	Personal Genomics

1

Introduction and Workshop Overview[1]

The completion of the Human Genome Project in 2003 was followed by the emergence of direct-to-consumer (DTC) genetic testing in 2006 and 2007, as companies such as 23andMe, Navigenics, and deCODE Genetics were founded. Companies attempting to market their products as health products directly to consumers met regulatory and clinical challenges. During that time, DTC companies could perform genetic testing for anywhere from $400–$1,000, making the price out of reach for many consumers. Today, the prices for such services are much lower, making DNA sequencing more accessible to consumers than before and providing opportunities for consumer health and literacy engagement. Additionally, DTC testing has had implications for clinical care, research, and education.

Consumer genomics, which includes both DTC applications (i.e., genetic testing accessed by a consumer directly from a commercial company apart from a health care provider) and consumer-driven genetic testing (i.e., testing ordered by a health care provider in response to an informed patient request) has evolved considerably over the past decade. In that time, DTC genetic testing has moved from more personal utility-focused applications outside of traditional health care, such as exploring ancestry, to interfacing

[1]The planning committee's role was limited to planning the workshop, and the Proceedings of a Workshop was prepared by the workshop rapporteurs as a factual summary of what occurred at the workshop. Statements, recommendations, and opinions expressed are those of individual presenters and participants and are not necessarily endorsed or verified by the National Academies of Sciences, Engineering, and Medicine, and they should not be construed as reflecting any group consensus.

with clinical care in non-traditional ways, such as collaborations between DTC companies and health systems.

As consumer genomics has increasingly intersected with clinical applications, discussions have arisen about the need to demonstrate clinical and analytical validity and clinical utility because of the potential for consumers to misinterpret the results of these tests and for ensuring the accuracy of the information for medical decision-making. Determining the clinical utility of consumer genomics entails examining the benefits and harms, which depend on various factors such as the availability of comparable risk assessment tools, costs of the intervention, and the personal value of the information (Khoury et al., 2009). In addition, the clinical readiness for and interest in this information have presented educational and training challenges for providers. Surveys of physicians have indicated that many of them are not confident in their ability to use genetic testing results in their patient care—a challenge for clinical genetic testing too (Owusu Obeng et al., 2018). At the same time, consumer genomics has emerged as a potentially innovative mechanism for thinking about health literacy and engaging participants in their own health and health care.

One of the reasons for using consumer genomics is its personal utility, or the usefulness that an individual derives from knowing his or her genetic information. If consumers are engaged and empowered to learn more about their health information and potential genetic risk factors, there could be opportunities for the health care system to learn effective strategies for engagement with consumers, including engaging populations that may not have adequate access to genetic testing. While the regulatory process for DTC genetic health risk tests involves the submission of a user comprehension study, there may still be questions about the extent to which consumer genomics companies are responsible for ensuring that consumers fully understand the information being presented to them so that they make informed decisions (Allyse et al., 2018).

The use of consumer genomics could also have implications for genetic research, given that many consumer genomics companies share participant data with external researchers for research and development purposes. To date, many of the individuals in genetic research studies and genomic databases are of European descent, meaning that data from underrepresented populations are lacking (Landry et al., 2018). If DTC genetic testing is able to reach traditionally underserved populations, data from consumer genomics companies may provide the opportunity to diversify datasets and help researchers gain more insights into the role that genetic differences play in individuals of different ancestry.

OVERVIEW OF THE WORKSHOP

To understand the complexity of the issues presented above more fully and to explore the current landscape of consumer genomics and the implications for how genetic test information is used or may be used in research and clinical care, the Roundtable on Genomics and Precision Health of the National Academies of Sciences, Engineering, and Medicine hosted a public workshop on October 29, 2019, in Washington, DC.[2] Discussions included such topics as the diversity of participant populations, the impact of consumer genomics on health literacy and engagement, knowledge gaps related to the use of consumer genomics in clinical care, and regulatory and health policy issues such as data privacy and security. A broad array of stakeholders took part in the workshop, including genomics and consumer genomics experts, epidemiologists, health disparities researchers, clinicians, users of consumer genomics research applications, representatives from patient advocacy groups, payers, bioethicists, regulators, and policy makers.

The idea for this workshop, explained Cathy Wicklund, the director of the graduate program in genetic counseling, an associate professor at the Feinberg School of Medicine's Center for Genetic Medicine at Northwestern University, and the workshop planning committee co-chair, grew out of a 2018 workshop on disparities in access to genomic medicine which raised the issue of whether some populations were missing the potential benefits of genomic medicine (NASEM, 2018). One of the things that the roundtable had looked at during those discussions was access to genetic services including genetic testing, and DTC genetic testing was seen as an area where individuals were accessing genetic services outside of the traditional public health or health care system model. This, Wicklund said, prompted the roundtable to explore how well companies are reaching diverse or underserved populations and if the opportunity exists to work with DTC service providers to decrease inequities and disparities in genomic databases and their applicability to underserved populations. Excluding newborn screening, it is possible that more people have had some form of genomic testing outside of the traditional health care model than within health care, said Greg Feero, a professor in the Department of Community and Family Medicine at the Geisel School of Medicine, a faculty member with the Maine Dartmouth Family Medical Residency Program, an associate editor for *JAMA*, and the workshop planning committee co-chair. As of 2018, consumer genomics industry estimates indicated that more than 12 million individuals had submitted samples for DTC genetic testing; by early 2019,

---

[2]The workshop agenda, speaker biographical sketches, Statement of Task, and registered attendees can be found in Appendixes A, B, C, and D, respectively.

MIT Technology Review estimated that 26 million people had contributed their DNA sequencing information to one of the large consumer genomics databases and that AncestryDNA and 23andMe were among the largest in terms of participants (Regalado, 2019).

The age of DTC genomics began 1 year before the first iPhone appeared, noted Geoffrey Ginsburg, the director of the Duke Center for Applied Genomics & Precision Medicine; a professor of medicine, pathology, and biomedical engineering at the Duke University Medical Center; and the roundtable co-chair. In the intervening 13 years, the concept of consumer genomics and DTC genomic testing has evolved considerably. While many have applauded the growing use of DTC genomics as an approach to thinking about how to engage the public in health literacy and their own health and health care, that sentiment is not universal, Ginsburg said. The clinical provider community, he continued, has worried about the day when patients start coming to their appointments with their genomic data and asking what the results mean.

In addition, there are some concerns that consumers are availing themselves of these tests without a clear picture of what information they provide and what other purposes their data may be used for, an issue that the workshop would examine in one of the panel sessions. Over the course of the workshop, Ginsburg said, "we are going to have an opportunity to look at the landscape of this continually evolving field and think about the implications for research, for clinical care, for reaching and giving access to the underserved and underrepresented communities." In addition, the workshop focused on health-related information coming from DTC testing, rather than ancestry insights, and considered the seminal question of how to integrate data from consumer genomics tests into health care.

SETTING THE STAGE: THE EVOLUTION OF DIRECT-TO-CONSUMER GENETIC TESTING

DTC genetic testing encompasses four major areas, explained Robert Nussbaum, the chief medical officer at Invitae and the opening keynote speaker at the workshop: ancestry; personal traits; multifactorial genetic risk scores for diseases such as type 2 diabetes, rheumatoid arthritis, and Crohn's disease; and testing for Mendelian disorders such as cardiomyopathy and hereditary breast and ovarian cancer. The use of DTC genomic tests by individuals to obtain information about their ancestry and personal traits can serve as a gateway to involving these people in research, though there is concern about the clinical utility of multifactorial genetic risk scores. For example, one study of relatives of people with Crohn's disease found that providing them with genetic test results had no effect on their smoking behavior, even for those relatives with elevated genetic risk scores for Crohn's disease (Hollands et al., 2012; Whitwell et al., 2011). Another review found that communicating genetic-based risk estimates had a similar lack of effect on health behavior changes for different multifactorial conditions where lifestyle modifications could be indicated (Hollands et al., 2016).

For Mendelian disorders, the value of DTC genomic testing depends to some extent on what type of analysis has been performed on an individual's genome. One type of analysis, for example, looks at individual genomic variants. Data from one unpublished study at Invitae that Nussbaum described showed that a 24-variant screen for familial hypercholesterolemia missed up to two-thirds of individuals whose whole-genome sequence identified a mutation in the low-density lipoprotein receptor gene involved in familial hypercholesterolemia. If someone is having DTC testing done for a different reason, such as ancestry, adding a medically relevant test in that setting can identify some healthy people who are not aware they have a potentially deleterious mutation, Nussbaum said.

In another unpublished study of more than 270,000 patients referred by health care providers for gene testing based on personal or family history of cancer, Nussbaum and his colleagues found that when they stratified the data by self-reported ethnicity, the test for one particular gene associated with a higher incidence of colorectal cancer, *MUTYH*, was 100 percent incomplete for Asians, which means, he said, the existing allele-specific DTC test for *MUTYH* mutations is not designed to test for any of the cancer-associated *MUTYH* variants found in Asians. Similarly, he said, the current test is 75 percent incomplete for African Americans, 46 percent incomplete for Latinos, and 33 percent incomplete for Caucasians. "Variant-specific DTC [panels], depending on what gene and what variant you're talking about, can have very different yields, depending on the ethnic background of the people involved," Nussbaum said.

The routes to obtaining genetic testing include the traditional health care provider-initiated service, DTC with no physician involvement, and hybrid models that are consumer-driven, but with physician involvement (Phillips et al., 2019) (see Figure 1-1). A hybrid model may be useful if there are roadblocks to accessing clinically valid genetic testing, Nussbaum said; such potential roadblocks include a scarcity of genetic counselors that leads to long wait times, the discomfort that non-genetics specialists may have in ordering a test, out-of-date testing guidelines, the cost of testing, the reluctance of insurers to pay for testing, and logistical barriers that DTC companies have been good at lowering. The hybrid model, he continued, engages with and does not ignore providers, and it limits the gatekeeping role of payers because consumers can order and pay for these tests directly. Nussbaum noted, though, that genetics specialists may still not like the hybrid model.

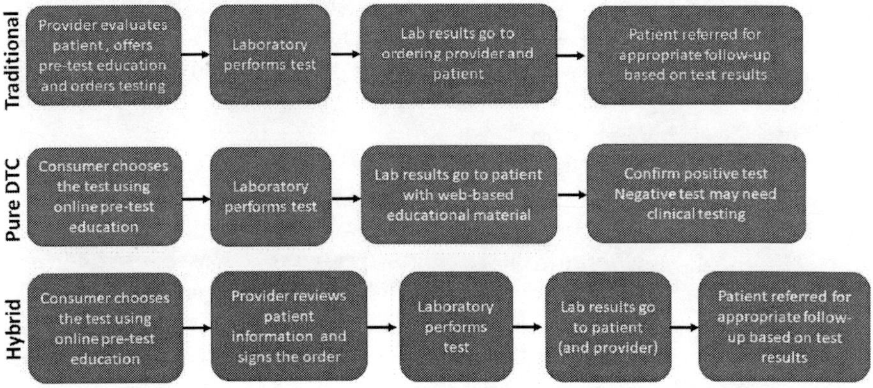

FIGURE 1-1 Models for genetic risk screening and testing.
SOURCE: Robert Nussbaum workshop presentation, October 29, 2019.

A survey of consumer attitudes toward the pure DTC and hybrid models that Nussbaum and his colleagues conducted found that diagnostic testing was the number one reason for having a test; 52 percent of the respondents gave this reason, compared with 49 percent who said they had a test to obtain ancestry and heritage information. Other common responses were pre-symptomatic and predictive reasons, proactive health testing, carrier testing, and non-health-related self-exploration. Consumers do have "paradoxical concerns" regarding genomic risk screening by this hybrid model, Nussbaum said, which makes it different from the pure DTC model. For example, respondents raised privacy concerns related to physician involvement and about the resulting clinical grade assigned to the results, which for many comes with a heightened sense that getting the test is a serious action. As a result, consumers have misperceptions about actionability and reservations about taking this kind of genetic test that stem from worries about the psychological burden of obtaining distressing information, he said.

Many consumers are also skeptical about the credibility and quality of the results—something Nussbaum calls the "Theranos effect"—given that payers will not cover these tests. At the same time, some consumers view keeping their genomic information private from insurers as a potential benefit of this model compared with the traditional physician-ordered model.

Consumers also voice real fears about several recurring issues, Nussbaum said. These include

- a general fear of having their genetic information existing "out there" in the ether;

- worries about identifying preexisting conditions their insurance will not cover or that will cause their premiums to increase;
- concerns that the testing company will sell their genetic data to unauthorized third parties;
- worries about government or law enforcement agencies gaining access to their data; and
- concerns about "bad actors" using their data for nefarious purposes.

In conclusion, Nussbaum said, a number of interesting paradoxes are found at the intersection among hybrid testing, the pure DTC, and the medical care system. "There is obviously a thirst for this information, yet people are not quite sure how best to get it," he said. "You would think they would be more reliant on their own physicians for it, and yet, I think there is some concern." In his experience, he said, consumers have a wide range of opinions and attitudes about genomic testing, so this should be taken into account when discussing what the "consumer" wants from or thinks about DTC testing.

2

Understanding Consumer Genomics Use

Important Points Highlighted by Individual Speakers

- Direct-to-consumer (DTC) genomic test purchasing is trending upward and may be moving toward a model where more individuals will undergo genetic testing outside of the traditional medical model than inside it, which means that health systems and providers will need to be prepared to help patients navigate the results from DTC genomic tests. (Bloss)
- The gap between patients believing they have the right to access genomic information without their physician and believing that their physician should be available to provide guidance creates an opportunity for developing methods and training for providers to better manage provider–patient interactions focused on DTC genomic test results. (Bloss)
- There are consistent consumer motivations for using DTC genomic tests across the literature, but more data are needed to better understand what effects there may be on individual behavior change as a result of undergoing DTC genetic testing. (Bloss)
- Resources that support psychological and emotional health should be available for individuals who experience significant psychological distress after receiving their DTC test results. (Bloss)

- Genetic counselors are important for helping patients understand the information produced by DTC genomic tests, the limitations of those tests, and what the next steps should be, given the specific test results. (Altschule, Pomerantz)
- Each consumer experience with DTC genomic testing is unique and therefore a more individualized approach for returning results may be necessary. (Altschule, Pomerantz)
- DTC genomic testing can be empowering for consumers and their families by giving them actionable information regarding current and future health risks. (Altschule)
- Receiving the results of a positive genetic mutation from a DTC genomic test should occur in the presence of a knowledgeable health care provider (e.g., a genetic counselor) rather than alone via email. (Pomerantz)

The workshop's first session, moderated by Tina Hesman Saey, a senior writer and molecular biology reporter for *Science News*, explored how consumers are engaging—or are not engaging—with direct-to-consumer (DTC) and consumer-driven genomics services and whether there are lessons to learn about overall health engagement. This session also provided insights into how patients and providers are using genomic data obtained through consumer genomics applications along with information from other sources to make health care–related decisions. Cinnamon Bloss, an associate professor in the psychiatry and family medicine and public health departments at the University of California, San Diego, spoke about the history and future of consumer genomics use. Then Sara Altschule, a freelance writer for *Bustle* magazine, and Dorothy Pomerantz, a managing editor at FitchInk, described their personal experiences after receiving results from DTC genomic testing.

EXAMINING THE HISTORY AND FUTURE OF CONSUMER GENOMICS USE

The story of DTC genomics has captivated both scientists and the public since its appearance shortly after the completion of the Human Genome Project in 2003, Bloss said. She mentioned some of the challenges that the field has experienced since its inception, particularly regarding regulatory permissions to offer health-related testing (see Figure 2-1). In terms of consumer use, she said, the decreasing cost of DTC testing as well as the increasing market value for DTC companies led to an increased number of consumers purchasing DTC genomic tests. It has been estimated that the market value for DTC genomic testing in 2010 was $10 million (Wright

2003	Human Genome Project complete
2006	**23andMe founded, controversy and debate about pros/cons**
2007	Navigenics founded
2008	TIME names retail DNA test (23andMe) invention of the year
2009	30 companies offering DTC tests
2010	**Estimated ~\$10 million market**
2010	Pathway announces Walgreens partnership to sell in stores
2010	GAO report released on July 22
2011	AMA letter to FDA suggesting all genetic testing involve a physician
2013	FDA issues notice to cease and desist
2015	FDA approves 23andMe Bloom Syndrome test
2016	Beginning of DTC genetic test inflection point
2017	**Estimated ~\$600 million global market value**
2017	**23andMe claims > 2 million consumers**
2017	April 6, FDA approves 23andMe risk test for 10 diseases/conditions
2017	Among leading companies, total consumers > 12 million
2018	FDA grants 23andMe marketing authorization for BRCA tests
2018	GlaxoSmithKline invests \$300 million in 23andMe for drug development
2018	**Estimated ~\$830 million global market value for DTC genetics**
2019	**Total number of consumers projected at > 26 million**
2021	MIT Tech Review predicts ~100 million customers
2025	Global DTC genetics market predicted at > \$2.5 billion

FIGURE 2-1 The history of direct-to-consumer (DTC) genomics testing uptake.
SOURCE: Cinnamon Bloss workshop presentation, October 29, 2019.

and Gregory-Jones, 2010) but that by 2018 the estimated market value had risen to \$830 million (Ugalmugale, 2019).

To get an idea of the impact that DTC genomic testing has had on consumers, Bloss and her colleagues recently conducted a rapid review of the literature, finding 69 articles focusing on genetic health risk tests. One challenge in understanding consumer motivations is that about half of the published studies to date have been based on cohorts of consumers from only three studies: the Impacts of Personal Genomics (PGen) study (Krieger et al., 2016; Roberts et al., 2017), the Scripps Genomic Health Initiative (Bloss et al., 2010; Darst et al., 2014), and the National Institutes of Health Multiplex Initiative (Kaphingst et al., 2012). Because the participants in these studies were recruited a decade ago, they are likely to be early adopters on the standard bell-shaped curve of consumer-driven technology adoption, Bloss noted. The diffusion of innovations theory argues that adopters in each of the various categories—innovators, early adopters, early majority, late majority, and laggards—have different characteristics (e.g., late adopters tend to be more conservative) (Rogers, 1962). Because consumer genomics has moved from the early adopter phase to the early majority phase, existing studies may not accurately inform use by and impacts on the current consumers, Bloss said.

The literature review indicated that the participants in the cohort studies to date have been mostly white and of high socioeconomic status, Bloss said, and their primary motivations for testing have been learning about ancestry, health, and family health history or simply curiosity. Few studies, she said, have examined differences in motivations and outcomes as a function of demographic diversity, though one study did find that there were few differences in motivations as a function of race (Landry et al., 2017). Bloss noted, however, that the groups in that study were very small. Changes in health behavior (e.g., exercise, diet, smoking) were self-reported by about 25 percent of the participants, though studies using objective and validated measures of behavior find few or no changes (Gray et al., 2017). In the few studies where changes have been observed, she said it was difficult to determine the size of the effects and their duration. Another area where more research may be needed is in understanding whether there are behavior changes in individuals who receive positive *BRCA* results from DTC genomic tests because those tests were not on the market 10 years ago, Bloss said.

Critics of DTC genomic testing have raised concerns that consumers may experience adverse psychological reactions, such as anxiety and depression, after obtaining the results of their tests. Currently, Bloss said, there is little evidence that this concern is valid, though she added that for the small number of individuals who do experience adverse responses, the consequences may be significant (Oliveri et al., 2018). For that reason, she said, it is important to have resources available to help those individuals who do experience significant psychological distress after receiving their test results.

Researchers have also found that about one-third of consumers share their DTC genomic test results with at least one health care provider, usually the individual's primary care physician. Data on the characteristics of individuals sharing DTC data with their primary care physician are also inconsistent, Bloss said. The outcomes of sharing vary, but in general the result is that individuals are reassured by their providers more often than providers end up changing the way they manage their patients' health. Consumers, Bloss said, believe they have a right to access genomic information without involving their physicians but also that physicians should be available and able to provide counseling even though they did not order the tests. This can place a considerable strain on physicians, Bloss added, given estimates suggesting that there have been some 3.6 million instances of DTC data sharing with physicians in the United States while there are only 850,000 practicing physicians in the country.

Going forward, Bloss said, she expects consumer uptake to continue rising exponentially because companies are now engaging in aggressive and targeted marketing campaigns. One key implication is that advertising, combined with the low cost of obtaining DTC genomic testing, will drive purchasing until the market is saturated, whenever that might be. Because data on consumer trends are limited, she added, newer studies—for example, using social media strategies to identify trends in real time—may be needed to assess the influence of demographic factors and the effects of emerging issues.

The rise of DTC genomic testing is taking place against the backdrop of a broad and shifting consumer health landscape that expects patients to be more autonomous and that offers more DTC health products, such as heart rate monitors and hearing aids. In addition, there are evolving ideas about what it means to be an expert and about the extent to which people need expert knowledge. The implication here, Bloss said, is that consumers will increasingly seek after-the-fact physician guidance regarding genomic and other DTC health tests.

The upward trajectory of people being tested outside versus inside the medical model is part of a broader trend of consumer interest in DTC products and devices that is likely to continue, Bloss said. "I think it would be useful to learn about this phenomenon, how it occurs in the trenches between physicians and their patients. Develop and teach ways for physicians and patients to approach these interactions . . . and think of this as an opportunity to engage people."

CONSUMER PERSPECTIVES

"In everyone's life, there are numbers we always remember, such as your Social Security number, your address, and your phone number," Sara Altschule said, "and now, thanks to my 23andMe genetic health report, I now have another number I will never forget: 617DELT." That is the mutation in Altschule's *BRCA2* gene that increases her risk of developing breast and ovarian cancer during her lifetime. While estimates vary, studies suggest that between 27 and 84 percent of women with a *BRCA2* variant will develop breast cancer and 11 to 30 percent will develop ovarian cancer by age 70 (Kuchenbaecker et al., 2017). About 12.8 percent of women in the general population will develop breast cancer, and 1.3 percent will develop ovarian cancer in their lifetimes (Howlader et al., 2019).

Getting that news at age 30 was quite devastating, Altschule said, particularly because she was never expecting to receive this news in the first place. Her sister had given her a 23andMe kit as a holiday present, and the two siblings were excited to learn more about their ancestry. It was no surprise to her that her results showed she was 77.1 percent Ashkenazi Jewish. While viewing the report, she saw the option to add genetic health results for an additional fee, and curiosity prompted her to add that package to her report. Upon viewing the updated report, she was relieved to find that the only red flag was the possibility of being slightly sensitive to gluten. Six months later, she received an email from 23andMe informing her that the company had received Food and Drug Administration (FDA) approval for DTC genomic tests for cancer risk, which included testing for three *BRCA1* and *BRCA2* variants associated with an increased risk for breast and ovarian cancer in women and prostate cancer in men that are most common in people of Ashkenazi Jewish decent.

This was a startling revelation, Altschule said, because no one, not even her doctor, had ever told her about her increased risk. She called her mother and learned that there was no history of breast or ovarian cancer in her mom's family, although her father's cousin had battled breast cancer and died from ovarian cancer and also had a *BRCA2* mutation.

At 2:00 on a Sunday morning, Altschule logged into the 23andMe website to see the new results. "When I saw the words, 'one variant detected,' my heart sank," she recalled. In that moment, she felt anxiety, fear, and shock, and she spent the next several hours searching for every piece of information she could find, from Wikipedia pages to Facebook groups. By that Friday, after learning all that she could about what it meant to be *BRCA2* positive, she sat in the office of a genetic counselor hoping to hear that it was a false positive. That was not the message, however, and a subsequent blood test confirmed the 23andMe result.

Altschule said that after a week of scouring the Internet, having the genetic counselor's reassurance and perspective was important. "Knowing that my risk of developing breast cancer at age 30 was 10 percent, versus the very scary lifetime risk of 85 percent, was a much easier pill for me to swallow," Altschule said. Moreover, she learned that her risk of developing ovarian cancer was significantly decreased because she had been taking oral contraceptives and, furthermore, that she would not face the choice of whether to have preventive surgery to remove her ovaries until she was around age 45.

The options going forward were still not great, she recalled. One was to have a mammogram, breast magnetic resonance imaging, pelvic ultrasound and exam, and CA-125 blood test every 6 months. The other option was to have a preventive double mastectomy with reconstruction at that time and consider having her ovaries removed at age 45. "I always tell people having a double mastectomy was the easiest and toughest decision of my life," she said. Though she was worried about how the decision would affect her physical and mental well-being, after spending time researching and talking with her family and friends and other women who carry the same gene variant, she knew what she wanted to do. "I can easily say today I have zero regrets, and it was the best decision for me," Altschule said.

When asked if she would recommend genetic testing to others, Altschule tells others to make sure they really want to know the answer. "It is like opening Pandora's box," she said. "You cannot unsee the diagnosis and you cannot unknow the information," and the information can affect family members as well. In her mind, she said, her 23andMe results not only saved her life, but may save the lives of people in her family who now know they are also *BRCA2* positive. As the end of the day, Altschule said, she feels lucky. "I am a true believer that knowledge is power, and I have never felt more powerful."

Dorothy Pomerantz's story was similar to Altschule's in that she is Ashkenazi Jewish, too, with an aunt on her father's side who died of breast cancer. At one point in the past, she said, she had talked to her doctors about genetic testing, but none thought that her family history was significant enough to indicate the need for testing. When she decided to send a sample to 23andMe, she was expecting confirmation that she did not carry *BRCA* mutations, but the moment she looked at her results after quickly moving through the long tutorial included with them, her world stopped: she had a *BRCA1* mutation. This meant that her risk of developing breast cancer or ovarian cancer by age 70 was 40–87 percent and 16–68 percent, respectively (Kuchenbaecker et al., 2017). "In that moment my life changed," she said. "I stood there in my home office and I was stunned."

Her primary care physician connected her to a breast cancer specialist at Cedars-Sinai Hospital who saw her the following day and reiterated the need for confirmation testing before moving forward. A second test confirmed the 23andMe result, and after a long and reassuring conversation with her genetic counselor, she decided to have a preventive double mastectomy and have her ovaries removed. With two children and a supportive group of friends who were going through menopause, Pomerantz said it was an easy decision for her to make. The ability to be there for her children growing up and having years of relief was worth the short-term pain, she added.

Nearly 1 year later, Pomerantz said, she is healthy and grateful that she learned her *BRCA* status when she did. "I got information that I was able to act on, and while the surgeries were difficult, they were nothing like what those surgeries would have been if I had cancer," she said. At the same time, she was left with some ambiguous feelings about how she received the information. Working full time with two children, Pomerantz said, she would have been unlikely to seek genetic testing or take the time to see a genetic counselor because she was unware of her increased risk; on the other hand, getting the results via an email was a terrible experience. "In that moment," she said, "I felt confused and alone, and my mind immediately went to the worst places."

Pomerantz said she was lucky to get her doctor on the phone quickly before she "went too deep down the *BRCA* Google hole," as she put it, but she worries about the women who cannot get their doctors on the phone or who do not have doctors at all. Because about half of the women with a *BRCA* mutation have no family history of breast cancer, there may be many women who turn to 23andMe for other reasons and get surprising news with real consequences, as Pomerantz and Altschule did.

Moreover, 23andMe looks at three *BRCA* variants that are prevalent in individuals of Ashkenazi Jewish ancestry, only some of a much larger number of *BRCA* variants linked to breast and ovarian cancer, which means that many women stand to receive a "clean bill of health" that could be misleading. "This is not to say that 23andMe should not offer a health screen," Pomerantz said, "but when dealing with serious health issues, people need someone to walk them through it." She said that she wishes she had received her diagnosis from a person rather than from an email so that she could have had support in that moment.

The customer experience matters, and home genetic tests could be more valuable if they came with the opportunity to talk to a genetic counselor, Pomerantz said. Before deciding to have testing done by 23andMe, she said, she felt that she knew a lot about genetics, but being informed about genetics is not the same thing as being ready to handle the emotional impact of a diagnosis. "The information in these results are complicated and nuanced," she said, "and, as with every big health decision in our lives, we need people to help walk us through the dark."

DISCUSSION

Communicating Information with Family Members

Sharing information with family members can be challenging, one workshop participant said, asking Altschule and Pomerantz how they went about sharing their *BRCA* status with family members. Talking to her mother immediately was easy, Altschule said, but it was difficult to talk to her sister, who would have a 50:50 chance of also having the same *BRCA2* variant. She relied on her genetic counselor and her mother to help her come up with the right words to use. Working with a genetic counselor was also crucial for her in helping her understand the impact for her family, she added, as the counselor walked her through how that conversation with family members might go and the best approach for communicating information. Because the mutation was present on her father's side, she had to tell his brother about the results as well. Written information, she said, was helpful to have when talking with relatives. Altschule said that when her uncle took the information to his family practitioner, he was told he did not need to be tested because he was a man, despite the fact that he had three daughters and a son. "I just found it so upsetting that this was what his doctor told him," she said. It is an incorrect conclusion that men cannot transmit breast and ovarian cancer mutations, a participant added, and this is an area where many physicians do not properly counsel their patients.

Pomerantz told both of her parents and her brother about her results immediately, but she said there was no sense of alarm. She also told her cousins who have daughters, but no one in her family has opted to get tested despite the fact that she gave them vouchers for genetic testing at a reduced price that she had received from her genetic counselor. While Pomerantz herself does not necessarily understand that decision, she said that wanting to know has to be an individual choice. Age is important as well, Altschule added, saying that she was ready to hear that type of information at 30, but she may not have been at 21.

Asked whether there is literature on why people choose not to get testing, Bloss said that that some people feel they do not want to know and go through their lives worrying about possible consequences. She also cautioned that, given the trends in the types of consumers who have undergone testing, there could be a self-selection bias in terms of the literature on this to date.

Patient Resources and Support for Understanding Risk

One workshop participant asked whether it is difficult to find information about *BRCA* mutations online, and both Pomerantz and Altschule said that finding information was not the problem. Altschule cautioned that it is easy to go down the "rabbit hole," given the breadth of resources available online, when you do not have a person delivering the results and are viewing them for the first time at 2:00 a.m., but she added that one thing she noticed was missing from the online conversations were the experiences of women and men who had a gene mutation but did not yet have cancer. Pomerantz said that what was missing for her were the experiences of individuals receiving surprising information from at-home genetic tests.

Getting that information is going to be hard no matter how it is received, but having a knowledgeable person on the phone to walk through what the information means would be ideal, Altschule and Pomerantz agreed. Another challenge is that the knowledge base about genetics and risk is still early, Pomerantz added, and having a genetic counselor there to help is important. The DTC tests also have limitations, and that is an important part of what needs to be discussed, she added. Having information that is personalized would be helpful, Altschule said. She said she would have preferred to see the risk information based on her current age rather than staring at the 85 percent risk that showed up on her results page.

In terms of understanding risk, there may be a psychosocial piece that is missing, a workshop participant said. While DTC tests have to achieve a certain level of comprehension among consumers to be considered safe and effective, the idea of what the information may mean emotionally for the consumer at that time may also be important.

Data Privacy and Research

One workshop participant asked whether Pomerantz and Altschule were concerned about how their data would be secured and used. Initially, Pomerantz said, she was very concerned about the safety of her data and chose all of the privacy options 23andMe offered when signing up for the test. However, after she received the test results, she changed all those options because she felt she wanted to do everything she could to help others. "If doctors are going to be able to take my DNA and use it for research, then I want to make that as available to them as possible," she said. She also joined the All of Us Research Program[1] with the same idea in mind. Altschule said she did not put much thought into her decision to make all of her data available for research when she took her test, but now believes it was the right thing to do. Asked if they thought differently about researchers having access to their data versus a pharmaceutical company, both indicated that they did not view the uses differently and hoped that pharmaceutical research could ultimately help patients with *BRCA1* and *BRCA2* mutations as well. Both said their primary concern was that insurance companies might someday deny coverage because of their mutation status.

There may also be opportunities for using the data from the millions of consumers of DTC genomic tests. If those consumers agreed to share their data, Geoffrey Ginsburg said, you could create a virtual cohort that would be many times the size of the All of Us Research Program at a fraction of the cost. "I think something worth thinking about are the latent assets that the consumer industry has created that could actually catapult the science and research further than anyone has gone before," he added.

[1]For more information about the National Institutes of Health's All of Us Research Program, see https://allofus.nih.gov (accessed December 16, 2019).

3

Exploring the Role of Diversity and Health Disparities in Consumer Genomics

Important Points Highlighted by Individual Speakers

- The lack of diversity in genomics databases renders genomic test results less useful for underrepresented populations than for individuals of European ancestry due to the likelihood of uncertain or false positive or negative results. (Callier, Fullerton, Hutson)
- It would be beneficial to develop evidence standards for gene inclusion on multigene panels as a way of reducing the return of variants of uncertain significance. Consumer genomics companies should also be very transparent about the limitations of test result interpretation, particularly for underrepresented groups who are going to be affected disproportionately. (Fullerton)
- As direct-to-consumer (DTC) genomic test costs decline, there should be opportunities for improving communication, building trust, and developing better tools to serve underrepresented populations. (Callier)
- DTC genomic testing services could offer a way for underrepresented populations to benefit from the fruits of genomic medicine, but doing so will depend on having adequate datasets, effective communication, and access to downstream services. (Fullerton)

- DTC companies could work on adjusting algorithms and models to account for the overrepresentation of data from white populations. (Fullerton)
- By encouraging consumers to see themselves as a percentage of allegedly distinct ethnic groups, commercial DNA tests may re-inscribe notions of race and miscommunicate the complexity of ancestry. (Callier)
- The research on factors affecting the use of consumer genomics is still evolving, and currently there is very little information available about how rural and underserved populations are using these tests. (Hutson)
- DTC genomics tests may help reduce health disparities in underserved communities, but in order for that to happen there will need to be a balance among patient autonomy, clinical utility, ensuring patient safety, and technological innovation. (Hutson)
- There could be opportunities for collecting genetic and non-genetic data to better understand the joint role these play in an individual's risk of developing disease; however, more research is needed to develop the models that can integrate these data. (Tung)

The second session of the workshop focused on the current lack of diversity in genomics research and databases and the effect that this may have on health disparities. This session also examined whether consumer genomics applications are reaching diverse populations. Jacquelyn Taylor, a professor and the Vernice Ferguson Endowed Chair in Health Equity at the New York University College of Nursing and School of Medicine, moderated the session, which included presentations by four panelists and an open discussion. Joyce Tung, the vice president for research at 23andMe, discussed access to direct-to-consumer (DTC) genetic tests and participation in research. Malia Fullerton, a professor of bioethics and humanities at the University of Washington School of Medicine, addressed the skewed evidence base for consumer genomics and how this may affect underrepresented populations. The implications of genetic ancestry testing for diverse populations and the communication challenges around health risks was discussed by Shawneequa Callier, an associate professor of clinical research and leadership at The George Washington University School of Medicine and Health Sciences and a special volunteer with the Center for Research on Genomics and Global Health at the National Human Genome Research Institute. Sadie Hutson, the assistant dean of graduate programs and a professor of nursing at the University of Tennessee,

Knoxville, then explored how rural and underserved populations are engaging with genomics services.

CONSUMER ACCESS AND RESEARCH PARTICIPATION

There are several ways in which 23andMe is trying to make genetics more accessible to consumers, Tung said. The primary approach of the company has been to make the tests affordable, but an equally important step has been to make reports easy to understand. Toward that end, all written materials go through several rounds of internal testing and redesign to identify the key points that people need to take away from these reports. Internal testing has shown that there is greater than 90 percent comprehension of these key points across a wide demographic range, Tung said.

Making its tests available online and over the counter are additional ways in which 23andMe tries to broaden uptake, particularly for those individuals who may not have access to a clinical center that offers genetic testing or to providers who will order the genetic testing. Providing the kits and returning the results by mail can also help bring in individuals for whom privacy is a big concern.

At the time of the workshop, 23andMe had sold approximately 10 million kits, Tung said, and those ordering them have been primarily of European ancestry. While there is a fairly substantial cohort of Latinos, African Americans, and East and South Asians among the company's customers, Tung said that this group is smaller than would be expected based on U.S. demographics. The age distribution is bimodal, with one peak in the 30s and another in the 50s to 60s, and women are slightly more likely than men to participate. The 23andMe customer base skews toward those with a slightly higher income and more education than the average members of the U.S. population, Tung said, although there are a substantial number of individuals without a bachelor's degree who have been tested. Approximately 90 percent of 23andMe customers are in the United States.

Approximately 80 percent of 23andMe's customers consent to participate in research, Tung said, a figure that has been consistent through the company's history, even as the price of testing fell and the pool of customers grew more diverse. A theme frequently heard from 23andMe customers who participate in research is their desire to help other people, Tung said. Concerning research participation by ethnicity, there are some differences, but none of the differences are very large, she said; one difference is that East and South Asians participate slightly less than other ethnic groups. There are also few differences in research participation by age or sex.

It is well known that there is not enough diversity in human genetics research, Tung said, and 23andMe cannot provide information it does not have. While the company is trying to develop reports that represent non-

European populations, the reality is that more topics have been studied in European populations, so that is the data the company has available to share. The lack of diversity in genetics databases also affects polygenic risk scores[1] that use common variants because of the smaller sample sizes available for non-European populations, Tung said. Without more data from underrepresented groups, she explained, it is difficult to create models that perform well in all ethnicities. For example, 23andMe examined the performance of a type 2 diabetes model that it trained across all ethnicities and found it was still performing better in Europeans than in groups of other ancestries.

23andMe is working in several ways to increase diversity in its genomics research, Tung said. The first initiative the company developed is called the Global Genetics Project,[2] which involves reaching out and engaging with customers who have four grandparents from underrepresented countries. A second initiative, the Population Collaborations Program,[3] relies on partnerships around the globe to genotype people and develop reference populations from underrepresented communities. In addition, the company is investing in whole-genome sequencing of some of its African American and Latino customers as a means of improving its imputation panels that are used for research. Data from the African American sequencing study are now available through the National Institutes of Health's database of Genotypes and Phenotypes,[4] Tung said, and 23andMe welcomes academic collaborations.[5] 23andMe is also currently in talks to develop a partnership to create a large, non-European reference panel, Tung said.

Finally, the company is exploring novel methods for developing polygenic risk scores so that the data they do have can be better leveraged, both within and across populations, to develop better scores for non-Europeans. Recent work has shown that these meta-analytic methods are producing better results, Tung said, and the company will continue to try to increase the number of non-Europeans participating in genetics-based research.

---

[1]Complex traits, including many diseases, are determined by variations in multiple genes that have smaller effect sizes and act over time often in conjunction with environmental factors. The aggregate risk of an outcome such as developing a disease based on those DNA variants is referred to as a polygenic risk score (Sugrue and Desikan, 2019).

[2]To learn more about the Global Genetics Project at 23andMe, see https://www.23andme.com/global-genetics (accessed December 3, 2019).

[3]To learn more about 23andMe's Populations Collaborations Program, see https://research.23andme.com/populations-collaborations (accessed December 3, 2019).

[4]The database of Genotypes and Phenotypes was developed to hold and share the data and results from studies that examine the relationship between genotype and phenotype in humans. The database can be accessed at https://www.ncbi.nlm.nih.gov/gap (accessed December 6, 2019).

[5]Information about research collaborations with 23andMe can be found at https://research.23andme.com/collaborate (accessed January 3, 2020).

DIVERSITY AND THE POTENTIAL FOR DISPARITIES

There is a skewed evidence base in human genomics research, and this matters for clinical genetic test performance and DTC genetic test performance, Malia Fullerton said. As a result of this skewed evidence base, she added, underrepresented populations are more likely to be affected, either from a lack of benefit because of uncertain results or from potential harms related to false positive or false negative results. Notwithstanding the ongoing efforts, Fullerton said, it is important to not wait for the evidence base to catch up to address this problem.

Awareness about DTC genomic testing varies across ethnic groups, Fullerton said, which suggests that improving the awareness of and access to DTC genomic testing would help address the currently recognized disparities in the uptake of these tests. However, she said, even if differences in awareness, education, marketing, and access were addressed in the near term, there would still be disparities in the clinical utility of DTC genomic tests. The reason, she added, is that the genomic research evidence base is markedly skewed toward individuals of northern and western European ancestry (Popejoy and Fullerton, 2016).

The vast overrepresentation of genomes from individuals of European ancestry in research databases matters to genomic discovery and translation because human populations vary genetically due to the evolutionary history of how humans dispersed across the planet, Fullerton said. Population differences become increasingly important when considering rarer variations—typically, gene variants with less than 1 percent minor allele frequency—that are exactly the sort of variation most likely to be involved in disease predispositions of high interest to precision medicine, she said.

As an example, the results of a study of 2,300 European Americans and 2,300 African Americans that was conducted by the National Heart, Lung, and Blood Institute's Exome Sequencing Project demonstrated that African Americans have, on average, a greater number of coding region variants than European Americans (Auer et al., 2016). In addition, a larger proportion of the rare variants were exclusive to African Americans than to European Americans in that study. Such differences suggest that when white and non-white individuals participate in DTC consumer genetic testing, particularly testing that focuses on the health impacts of rare genetic variation, the test results can vary in their quality and accuracy, even when exactly the same test is being used, Fullerton said.

There are different types of outcome disparities that can result from these evidentiary disparities. For example, given that sequence-based tests can detect variants that have not been observed previously and whose clinical significance is unknown, individuals who come from population genetic backgrounds that remain underrepresented in the current evidence database are more likely to receive uncertain genetic test results (Caswell-Jin et al., 2018).

Consumers from underrepresented backgrounds can be also be harmed by receiving results misclassified as pathogenic as a result of a failure to consider ancestry-matched controls in the course of variant interpretation, Fullerton said. For example, one retrospective analysis of patients who had undergone clinical genetic testing for a condition known as hypertrophic cardiomyopathy found that a number of variants initially returned as pathogenic were subsequently reclassified once data on their frequency in unaffected African ancestry individuals became available (Manrai et al., 2016). While there are fewer direct comparisons to draw on with regard to potential false negative findings, recent work that has been focused on the generalizability of polygenic risk scores, for example, suggests that scores which have been validated in European ancestry populations may be poor predictors of genetic risk in individuals from other ancestral genetic backgrounds (Martin et al., 2019).

For consumers, there is currently no obvious near-term remedy for these potential test outcome disparities, Fullerton said. The ability to obtain one's complete raw genotype data file as a direct download could, in theory, allow consumers to take their DTC genomic test results to a third-party interpretation service in an effort to identify additional information that was not available in the initial DTC genetic testing encounter, she said. The problem, she said, is that nearly all of these third-party interpretation tools draw on the same skewed genomics reference evidence base. Additionally, there are no good estimates of how many DTC genomic test customers actually choose to download their data and explore options for additional corroborations or interpretation. When one of Fullerton's recent projects surveyed more than 1,100 self-identified DTC genomic test customers, it found that 72 percent had downloaded their raw data file and taken it to a variety of third-party interpretation tools designed to provide information about health-related risks and ancestry (Nelson et al., 2019).

Regarding possible solutions, Fullerton said that DTC genomic testing services may be the easiest way in the near term for traditionally underrepresented populations, including those with uneven health care access or health insurance coverage, to benefit from the fruits of medical genetics and precision medicine. However, steps should be taken to ensure that disparities are not further exacerbated by continuing to use the same skewed data. In her opinion, she said, DTC genomic testing companies should consider exploring the use of analytic or algorithmic adjustment, a point that Tung had discussed earlier regarding the efforts at 23andMe to improve the predictive accuracy of polygenic risk scores. Having an awareness of biases in the genomics space is critical as new algorithms are designed that take into account the uneven nature of the data, Fullerton said.

The field should also consider adopting evidence standards for gene inclusion on multigene panels, Fullerton said, as a way of reducing the number of variants of uncertain significance that get returned to participants. At the same time, she said, there is a need to be more transparent to consumers about the limitations of test result interpretation, particularly for underrepresented groups whose members are going to be affected disproportionately by the problems she identified.

Ultimately, the ethnically skewed evidence base undercuts the value of all genetic testing, including DTC genomic testing, Fullerton said. Even with greater attention to access and education, underrepresented minority populations are going to benefit less often and more often be harmed as a consequence of these evidentiary biases, she said. "We need to be looking into the adoption of analytical approaches that can be implemented, even while we rectify the underlying data biases," she said. "These corrections are urgently needed and cannot wait until the evidence base becomes more diversified."

IMPLICATIONS OF GENETIC ANCESTRY TESTING FOR DIVERSITY AND COMMUNICATION ABOUT HEALTH RISKS

The 1977 television mini-series *Roots* inspired some African Americans to start asking deep, significant, and often painful questions about their ancestry and their past. In a way, Shawneequa Callier said, genetics-based ancestry testing has become a point of entry for African Americans into the consumer genomics marketplace. However, caution needs to be exercised to prevent overselling DTC ancestry tests as a way to identify exactly where someone's ancestors came from with precise geographic detail, she said. Furthermore, a recent advertising campaign from Ancestry designed to reach African Americans missed the mark, she said, and greater care and cultural sensitivity is required when reaching out to underrepresented, marginalized populations.

One problem with DTC ancestry tests serving as an entry point into the world of genetics for underrepresented populations is that consumers may not understand the complexity of genetic ancestry, Callier said (Royal et al., 2010). "By encouraging consumers to see themselves as a percentage of allegedly distinct ethnic groups, commercial DNA tests may re-inscribe notions of race and miscommunicate the complexity of ancestry," Callier said. "Furthermore, the validity of these tests has come into question, which could impede trust in the technologies and possibly spill over into the clinical genetics testing realm." For example, in 2019 investigators at *Consumers' Checkbook* sent DNA samples to three different DTC genomic testing companies, and the ancestry results for one African American staffer varied widely, ranging from 18 percent West African and 33 percent Central

African to 87 percent West African and 3 percent Central African (Brasler, 2019).

Another challenge for DTC ancestry tests lies in the inconsistent way in which ancestry is discussed by consumers and researchers alike, Callier said. For example, the term "continental ancestry" or the idea that someone descends from "African Ancestry" or "European Ancestry" populations obscures the tremendous amount of diversity that exists on those continents and within the associated populations. In fact, Callier said, there may be a missed opportunity to use consumer genomics as a new way to engage in discussions about ancestry. As to the question of whether genetic ancestry tests are improving the way consumers think about race, two studies have found that consumers pick and choose the genetic ancestries they want to embrace (Roth and Ivemark, 2018; Shim et al., 2018). In other words, she said, test results had no effect on how people perceived who they are or the communities and people with whom they affiliated.

Currently, it is not clear whether DTC genomic testing can be useful for engaging with African American populations and if these tests should be used in the clinical setting, Callier said. Some investigators say that ancestry tests misrepresent human genetic diversity, and they argue that these tests should not be used in the medical setting (Blell and Hunter, 2019). Others, including Fullerton, have recognized the potential that consumers will share and discuss genetic ancestry results with providers, for which providers must be prepared (Royal et al., 2010). There could be some potential value to DTC ancestry tests, Callier said, but it will be important as the field moves forward to bring clarity and consensus to the way that ancestry is discussed. A recent study of 10 clinical laboratories found that the labs were not providing the same descriptive categories to designate a group or population (Popejoy et al., 2018). Several groups have argued that it is time to rethink how ancestry is talked about and reported in the literature (Bonham et al., 2018; Cooper et al., 2018; Nelson et al., 2018).

As the cost of sequencing declines, improving genetic and genomic literacy, particularly among underserved populations, will be an important endeavor, Callier said. In closing, she asked, Are there missed opportunities for developing clear and concise language related to race, ethnicity, and ancestry and opportunities for building trust related to genetic and genomic testing services?

RURAL AND UNDERSERVED POPULATIONS AND ENGAGEMENT WITH GENOMICS SERVICES

"As more companies enter the direct-to-consumer retail market for genomics, the increase in numbers of genotyped consumers will allow for an exponential increase in innovation," Sadie Hutson said, "but this is only going to happen if the reach expands beyond individuals of European descent." The analysis of rare variations, she explained, becomes much more powerful when sample sizes increase and become more diverse.

Echoing previous speakers in this session, Hutson described the under-representation of non-European, rural, and underserved populations in genomic databases as problematic, as it creates bias in foundational databases that exacerbates disparities. The result is that clinical interventions, polygenic risk scores, and guidelines for risk reduction and the management of complex chronic diseases may be largely inaccurate, particularly for diverse populations (Wojcik et al., 2019).

To provide some background about rural and underserved populations and their engagement with genomic services, Hutson described a 2016 study of a rural community in West Virginia in which more than half of the participants reported a high interest in participating in genetics and genomics studies to improve health (Mallow et al., 2016). Many of the individuals, the study found, were concerned about the influence of environmental health, including how exposure to harmful substances may be changing their genomes. This concern, Hutson said, was frequently cited by patients in her own practice in eastern Kentucky, where coal mining remains a major industry.

The participants in Mallow's study were divided in their attitudes, with some reporting little fear of the risks of genetics studies, while others cited a fear of the unknown, which can be a barrier to pursuing genetic testing. Other barriers that the participants reported included their concerns that knowledge about disease risk would not actually translate into action to prevent disease occurrence and that they mistrusted or had low confidence in their health care providers' knowledge about genetics and genomics.

Hutson said that the factors affecting the uptake of consumer genomics services that she sees regularly in her practice include a lack of awareness of DTC genomics testing (Salloum et al., 2018; Sussner et al., 2009; Vadaparampil et al., 2006), a lack of awareness about genetic counseling, and a lack of access to genetic counseling (Fogleman et al., 2019) (see Box 3-1). It is important to recognize, she said, that the literature on factors affecting the use of consumer genomics is still evolving, with little knowledge at present that is specific to rural and underserved populations.

Cost is one of the most frequently cited barriers affecting the use of DTC genomics testing services. In a survey by the Personalized Medicine Coalition (Personalized Medicine Coalition, 2018) of more than 1,000 American adults over the age of 18, 25 percent of those surveyed said they would willingly pay $50 to $100 for such services, but 30 percent were unwilling to pay any amount out of pocket. The respondents also mentioned privacy concerns, and only 10 percent said their provider had ever talked to them about genetic testing to diagnose a disease or guide

BOX 3-1
Factors Affecting the Use of Consumer Genomics Services (as presented by Sadie Hutson)

- Lack of awareness of direct-to-consumer (DTC) services
  - Awareness of DTC is lower among rural residents and racial and ethnic minorities
  - Awareness of genetic testing can vary by acculturation and by racial and ethnic identity
- Lack of awareness of genetic counseling
- Lack of access to genetic counseling
- Cost
- Privacy concerns
- Differences in discussions about genetic testing by health care providers
- Sociodemographic factors
- Family communication
- Fear of discrimination
- Barriers can change over time

treatment. A 2012 literature review found that a majority of consumers preferred receiving guidance from a health care provider regarding the use of DTC genomic tests (Goldsmith et al., 2012).

Family communication is generally very important to individuals in rural areas, Hutson said, and it can have both a positive and negative influence on discussions about genetics and family history. “While the number one reason for participating in genetic testing is to learn information for family members, concerns about guilt or fear of passing on genetically linked health conditions can be a major deterrent for testing,” she said. While fear and concerns about discrimination can be a barrier, Hutson said she has seen this factor decrease in importance for some populations in her practice. Many of the barriers to genetic testing and counseling in rural populations have been changing over time, she said.

Supporters of DTC genomics argue that this approach to genetic testing can benefit underserved populations, citing patient empowerment as the primary reason for that optimism, Hutson said. Other positive factors include the relative affordability of DTC testing, non-invasive sample collection, and increased accessibility to genetic testing. Increased patient engagement can lead to overall improvements in genetics literacy, Hutson said, but challenges remain, including the need to have DTC genetic testing results confirmed by more expensive methods which many patients may not be able to afford. As a result, she said, important decisions about treatment or disease management may be based on incomplete, inaccurate, or misunderstood information on the part of both the patient and the health care provider.

The availability of DTC genomics tests does not necessarily improve access for those who have existing barriers to access for general health care needs, Hutson said. In addition, there are privacy concerns about the unauthorized use of an individual's genomic data and about how such data will affect relatives. Wrap-around contracts[6] can result in consumers unknowingly consenting to terms and conditions regarding the privacy of their genetic data, Hutson said.

There are, however, opportunities to expand the reach of all types of genetic testing into underserved populations. In her own practice at the Pikeville Medical Center, Hutson said, she developed a cancer genetics program in which two genetics nurse navigators help patients complete family and personal health history information during a routine visit with the oncologist or over the phone. The navigators also provide an extensive overview of what will happen at their visit with Hutson, including providing background about her as someone who is not originally from the area, something that she found is important for improving trust with her patients. Patients are assisted in completing a three-generation family history questionnaire before meeting with Hutson. This pre-visit process with the navigators decreased the no-show rate for the cancer genetics service and increased patient encounters by 54 percent in 1 year, Hutson said. The workflow relies on the nurses, who come from the community, to provide background information on the patients before they are seen.

Hutson is also partnering with a nurse-led initiative called the Health Wagon, which provides high-quality care to medically underserved communities in southwest Virginia. Given the cancer disparities in this region, where 98 percent of the residents are uninsured and 70 percent live on less than $20,000 per year, many patients have a clinical indication for genetic testing, she said. To address the cost barrier, she partnered with Invitae, which provides free testing for all individuals referred by the Health Wagon, and she provides free genetic counseling. Telemedicine and faith-based initiatives can also serve as avenues for increasing the reach of and promoting accessibility to genetic testing, Hutson said.

Meeting people where they are and communicating with them in terms that are easily understood is important, Hutson shared. For example, Hutson does not use the term "genetic mutations," but rather "genetic changes," an easier and potentially less frightening concept to grasp. It is also critical to set aside enough time to truly work with individuals who come in with questions

[6]Wrap contracts, also called clickwrap or browsewrap contracts, are contractual agreements between a business and its consumers. These contracts are often available online and can be entered into with a single click.

about genetics. Ideally, Hutson said, she likes to spend 45 minutes with all new patients and 30 minutes for appointments at which she discloses and discusses test results. Spending enough time with each patient is of critical importance, Hutson said, and it requires a thorough review of all patient and family history information before the visit, which assures efficiency and the capacity to build trust with the patient. That trust is critical, especially if other family members need to be tested, she said.

Genomics-based test results, including those from DTC tests, can be confusing, particularly since different test services and providers may be providing conflicting information regarding specific test results. "In my experience, some providers may order testing and not provide results or provide misinformation or incomplete information about results to patients," Hutson said. Given that the landscape of genetic and genomic testing is evolving rapidly, efforts are needed to educate providers of all types and experience levels about these tests and the resources available for their practices and patients.

For DTC genomics tests to reduce disparities in underserved communities, there will need to be a balance between patient autonomy, clinical utility, ensuring patient safety, and technological innovation, Hutson said. Consumer genomics disintermediates the health care provider from the process of obtaining personal genetic information, but this approach may have broader implications related to medical management as well as psychosocial consequences for patients who decide to undergo DTC genetic testing, she said. There is a critical opportunity for multiple sectors to work together to ensure the proper inclusion of all individuals in genomic testing, she added.

DISCUSSION

Direct-to-Consumer Genomics Tests and the Social Determinants of Health

How, one workshop participant asked, can the results from DTC genomics tests be interpreted alongside the social determinants of health to give a more complete picture of one's health? 23andMe is interested in this issue, Tung said, yet the company is struggling with the fact that consumers want a unified score that integrates all of their risk factors, both genetic and environmental. However, the data and models to create that type of unified score do not exist yet, she said, and 23andMe is still in the early stages of collecting data and developing methods in this area. 23andMe's efforts are to be applauded, Fullerton said, but it is important to note that the majority of 23andMe's customers are white and well-educated and have higher incomes than the average American, so the information the company will gather to help predict the joint role of genes and the environment may only apply to the subset of people least affected by health disparities.

For example, Fullerton said, studying genetic variations in the *APOL1* gene, which can result in a higher risk of chronic kidney disease, is challenging in part because the variants are not fully penetrant. There is likely a role for the social determinants of health in the expression of the risk phenotype for chronic kidney disease in African Americans. Hutson agreed that further research is needed to better understand the relationship between a person's genes and his or her environment, and she cited as an example coal miners in rural areas who may be exposed to toxins.

Ancestry Testing as a Potential Entry Point for Underrepresented Populations into Genetic Testing

Another workshop participant asked about the potential benefits or harms of using ancestry testing as an entry point into the genetic testing market. The benefit of this approach, Callier said, is that it encourages individuals to engage in discussions about genetics and brings together families and communities to dig into historical archives and records about their history. The downside, she said, is that those in the ancestry testing market and medical community are failing underrepresented consumers in terms of the way they discuss race and ancestry. 23andMe's ancestry-only product was quite popular, Tung said, potentially because it was a softer introduction to genetics than thinking about health-related implications. As one example, a primarily African American community group in the San Francisco area partnered with 23andMe for ancestry testing. Following the test, the group held a lengthy open discussion with 23andMe in a town hall setting where they were able to ask questions and share information with one another. This type of engagement approach helped the company understand the community's concerns and build trust, Tung said, although she cautioned that it is important not to overgeneralize because this was just one specific example.

Fullerton said that in her study of customers of consumer genetic testing who had downloaded their raw data, that many of those individuals were initially interested in their ancestry, but subsequently became aware of the ability to use third-party interpretation services to learn about health-related information. This crosswalk between ancestry and health information also existed in the opposite direction, she noted, with individuals who sought consumer genetics testing initially for health information later wanting to know more about their ancestry.

Increasing Genetic and Genomic Literacy and Strengthening the Workforce

Panelists were asked if there is a role for the consumer genomics industry in efforts to increase genetic and genomic literacy and the diversity of the genomics workforce. 23andMe has educational materials it offers to high school teachers and college students to support genetics education and literacy, Tung said, but the company has not figured out how best to scale its efforts. There could also be opportunities for DTC genomics companies to partner with individuals and groups who are interested in education within their communities, Callier said, but this should not be a top-down effort. Those living in rural communities, Hutson said, need a great deal of help in terms of education about genetics and genomics. Starting with a needs assessment that informs a tailored educational approach for rural communities might be the best approach, she said.

It may be advantageous to bring community health workers into this effort both as a means of diversifying the workforce and as a means of forming stronger connections with the community, Fullerton said. These individuals are already working in the community, are trained to provide important health information, and could play a critical role in helping people understand the importance of family health history. Intersections between the DTC business community and the public health community have not been fully explored, she said, and it will require more work from both groups to make a meaningful difference.

4

Integration Within Scientific and Medical Communities

Important Points Highlighted by Individual Speakers

- Innovative data-sharing agreements and other collaborations with consumer genomics companies can enable high-quality, scalable genetic research for discovery. (Singleton)
- Both consumers and clinicians need to be informed about what it means, given the intricacies of the information and lack of clear treatment guidance, for tests to reveal variants of uncertain significance. (Dolan)
- Increase coverage of and access to genetic counseling by independently licensing and paying genetic counselors in each state. (Dolan)
- Long-term, sustained engagement of consumers can occur through creating verification programs, developing tools for health care providers, producing accessible and scalable genetic counseling, producing gene- and variant-specific reports, and updating reports with notifications. (Bonadies)
- Direct-to-consumer (DTC) testing creates an opportunity for people to talk about behaviors, habits, and practices that are important for their health; to engage with their providers; and to have meaningful conversations about genetics and genomics. (Ferber)

- Getting data from DTC test services into the electronic health record is still a challenge and will require setting some standards to enable integration. (Ferber)

The workshop's third session, moderated by Bruce Blumberg, a professor of clinical science and a planning co-lead of faculty development at the Kaiser Permanente School of Medicine, discussed factors that may affect how consumer genomics data are integrated into clinical care. The session's four panelists also examined the challenges of and opportunities for using consumer genomics data for research and explored emerging cross-sector collaborations and potential lessons to learn. Andrew Singleton, a senior investigator in the Laboratory of Neurogenetics at the National Institute on Aging, discussed how data from direct-to-consumer (DTC) genomic tests can help inform research on the genetics of complex diseases. Siobhan Dolan, a professor and the vice chair for research in the Department of Obstetrics and Gynecology and Women's Health at the Albert Einstein College of Medicine, spoke about work to integrate genetics and genomics into clinical care. Danielle Bonadies, the director of genetics at My Gene Counsel, addressed different paths to integrating DTC test result data into the medical model of disease. And Matthew Ferber, an associate professor of laboratory medicine and pathology and a consultant to the Division of Laboratory Genetics and Genomics in the Department of Laboratory Medicine and Pathology at the Mayo Clinic, discussed the lessons his institution has learned from its work on what he called a "near-consumer" testing experience.

INCORPORATING DIRECT-TO-CONSUMER DATA INTO COMPLEX DISEASE RESEARCH

Singleton reviewed some recent work in which he and his colleagues, in collaboration with 23andMe, examined genome-wide associations to identify genetic variants associated with Parkinson's disease (Nalls et al., 2019). His group started investigating common genetic variability in Parkinson's disease in 2005 and have identified 90 individual risk factors that increase the odds of developing this disease. This work required large sample sets, such as the population-scale cohorts of the UK Biobank and 23andMe's growing cohort of individuals with Parkinson's disease and controls. The group began working with 23andMe around 2011, and in a meta-analysis that year 23andMe participants accounted for approximately 3,400 out of the study's 15,000 patients with Parkinson's disease and approximately 29,600 out of 50,000 total controls, Singleton said (Do et al., 2011; IPDGC and WTCCC2, 2011). By 2019, 23andMe participants accounted for approximately 13,000 out of 37,700 patients with the disease and approximately 935,000 out of 1.4 million total controls, he added (Nalls et al., 2019). 23andMe participants currently account for one-third of the cases that Singleton's group studies and 70 percent of its control group. Without those cases, Singleton said, he and his group would most likely not have learned of about 30 to 40 important genetic loci in Parkinson's disease. Driven by a common interest, 23andMe and Singleton's team are now looking for genetic associations between Parkinson's disease and other traits and also seeking to determine whether the genetic basis for this disease differs between men and women.

Though some have questioned the quality of the data from DTC genomic testing services, Singleton said that, in his experience, the data are of the same quality as the data his group generates at the National Institutes of Health. In addition, he said, 23andMe has been quite responsive when it comes to sharing or analyzing data, perhaps because of the involvement of foundations and other philanthropic organizations. One issue that does arise has to do with not contravening any work the company is engaging in with corporate clients. The work that Singleton's group does with the company has to be non-competitive with the work of 23andMe's corporate partners. Another issue is that some types of data are not easily accessible, and current policy limits broad data-sharing agreements. For example, Singleton's group never sees 23andMe's raw data, only summary statistics, and anyone who wants those data after his group publishes its work has to engage in a separate data agreement with 23andMe. However, the company does have a clear and effective process for requesting data, he added. In terms of scale, some 7 million to 8 million people have been genotyped in the cohort being studied, with about 20,000 Parkinson's disease patients in that cohort.

There are other ways that these data are being used in research, Singleton said, such as a project being conducted with The Michael J. Fox Foundation for Parkinson's Research and 23andMe. In this project, individuals with Parkinson's disease can upload reams of information about themselves to the Fox Insight web portal, including their electronic health records, diaries of daily activities, and genomic test results from 23andMe.[1] The patients' data belong to the individuals, but they are also available for researchers to use. "This is a neat research idea, and one that I am surprised has not been used more often," Singleton said.

A relatively new company, LunaDNA, also has a web portal for individuals to contribute their genomic test data and health care information, Singleton said.[2] In return, everyone who contributes data receives a

[1]For more information about Fox Insight, see https://foxinsight.michaeljfox.org (accessed December 11, 2019).

[2]For more information about LunaDNA, see https://www.lunadna.com (accessed December 11, 2019).

small ownership interest in the company. When researchers pay to conduct research on the de-identified and aggregated data, the proceeds are passed along to those who shared their data. "I do not know if this will work," Singleton said, "but I think it is an interesting concept in terms of thinking about ownership of data and patients or individuals taking control and making use of their own genetic data." One participant asked how researchers can account for DTC data coming from a database like LunaDNA if they are also collecting data from a DTC company. In his laboratory, Singleton said, a check sum is created, which provides information about genetic identity that is cross-referenced with the check sum number coming from the DTC company. In that way, any duplicate individuals can be removed.

INTEGRATING GENETICS AND GENOMICS DATA

As a physician in the Bronx, Siobhan Dolan said, she provides care to a diverse and vibrant community of more than 1.4 million citizens. Almost 60 percent of this population speaks a language other than English at home, more than 30 percent live in poverty, and 10 percent do not have health insurance, yet more than 80 percent of households in the Bronx have a computer at home. The Department of Obstetrics and Gynecology and Women's Health at the Montefiore Medical Center has a team of 7 genetic counselors and 3 clinical geneticists who together see between 30 and 40 patients per day. The patients include those undergoing prenatal genetic testing, cancer patients, and those seeking care for other reasons, such as multiple miscarriages and infertility. In her experience, Dolan said, she does not have patients coming to see her with their DTC genomic test results, although there are other patient-driven, non-medical concerns related to genetic testing that she sees as a clinician.

Prenatal genetic testing can provide expectant parents with a great deal of information, including aneuploidy diagnosis and carrier status, Dolan noted, but she added that what many patients are really interested in is the sex of their child. The gender reveal phenomenon,[3] she said, creates a complicated paradigm for clinical care because the person taking the test often does not want to receive the results personally and because expecting parents want the results early in order to plan their gender reveal party. The problem with this, she said, is that people sometimes enter into prenatal genetic testing with little consideration that they might also receive the results of high-risk genetic screening tests, despite having gone through the informed consent process prior to testing.

[3]For a brief background on "gender reveal parties," see https://www.washingtonpost.com/news/parenting/wp/2018/05/13/how-do-parents-find-out-the-sex-of-their-baby-today-exploring-the-new-trend-of-gender-reveal-parties (accessed December 13, 2019).

Another challenge is the lack of integration of genomic test results into an individual's electronic health record, Dolan said. As a result, test results are not easily accessible by the patient through a web portal, and patients cannot get the information they want. Given the challenges with the patient interface, patients can sometimes misinterpret a fragile X screening result for the gender as well. Paternity testing is another element that patients are interested in, although Dolan said that this is not something her clinic does because it falls under a legal, not medical, model. Nonetheless, many patients inquire about paternity testing and wonder whether DTC genetic testing can be used to establish paternity. From her perspective, Dolan said, there can be a lot of consequential family structure information to consider. Sometimes patients will also request amniocentesis in order to determine paternity, which can be ethically challenging for providers.

A question that arises with cancer genomics is how to connect the high-risk patients, those who need genetics or genomics services, with their department. On occasion, for example, individuals will come in with a list of relatives, each of whom had a different cancer when they were in their 80s, and they are worried about their risk of developing cancer. Dolan said that in such a situation she will explain that the pattern does not fit a pattern of genetic risk. In other cases, she sees individuals diagnosed with breast or ovarian cancer who have a strong family history of those cancers and regrets the missed opportunity to find those individuals early, before they developed cancer. Obtaining important information from family members can be further complicated by the challenges in finding and accessing old test results and family health history information. Family members may not remember the results and therefore may inadvertently convey incorrect information.

Patients are often interested in multigene panels and in learning as much as they can about their genetic risk factors, Dolan said. She talks to patients about variants of uncertain significance before ordering the test so that they are not blindsided when they receive their test results. As a provider trying to communicate uncertainty, she said, it can be challenging to explain the complexities of variants of uncertain significance in a way that patients can really understand. Many patients are very interested in how to use the information they receive, but when Dolan explains that uncertainty is complex and that there are not necessarily clear guidelines for how to interpret that information, her patients will often try to find utility in in spite of that, and say, for example, that they will eat better and exercise more.

While much of the focus in consumer genomics is on helping increase consumers' understanding, Dolan said that there are various challenges relating to providers as well. For example, she mentioned a surgeon wanting to operate based on a variant of uncertain significance. Risk is a continuum where the evidence is constantly evolving, and really understanding the intricacies of genetic test results is quite complicated, Dolan said.

INTEGRATING DIRECT-TO-CONSUMER DATA INTO THE MEDICAL MODEL OF DISEASE

Given the current estimates of DTC genomic testing services, an average of about 42,000 people undergo testing every day, Danielle Bonadies said, and by 2021 about 100 million Americans—one-third of the U.S. population—are expected to have had their genomes analyzed by one of these services. What that means, she said, is that whether a given individual had a DTC test, at least one relative of that individual will likely have had a DTC test (Khan and Mittelman, 2018). "Therefore," she said, "some of your data, by being genetically related, is in that database."

Bonadies said that she has seen in her clinic that patients have many residual questions after getting the results of their tests, such as what the tests did and did not look for, what they need to do next with the information from the tests, and how the information will affect the management of their health. On social media, she said, there are discussions about the accuracy of these tests and attempts to correct misinformation about positive and negative results. In some cases, the DTC model is merely transactional—send in a sample, get results—with little discussion about family history, verification testing, risk, medical management, or long-term care and surveillance.

A major question is how to integrate the data from DTC testing into the medical model so that an individual's providers can access the data and help the individual understand what the data mean. One path, Bonadies said, could be through verification testing, where the verified results are integrated into the electronic health record. In one study of just under 50 patients, verification testing found that 40 percent of the results were false positives and that 19 percent were confirmed but classified inaccurately as pathogenic by the DTC service (Tandy-Connor et al., 2018). What was not examined in this study but that has been looked at by other investigators is how many positives DTC testing would have identified in individuals with a strong personal or family history of breast, ovarian, or colon cancer. The results, which have not yet been published, Bonadies said, showed that between 80 and 90 percent of the associated genetic markers would not have been picked up on a DTC genomics test, indicating that some consumers may be missing potentially important health information.

Despite the limitations, there are still routes for incorporating the significant and valid information that DTC genomic tests can produce, Bonadies said. Her company, My Gene Counsel, is building a bridge from DTC testing into medical-grade testing and the medical system by offering genetic counseling and verification testing to individuals who have received a DTC finding or individuals who have concerns about their personal or family medical history. If those individuals are candidates for genetic testing and counseling, the company will help them navigate those routes. Several insurers, including Blue Shield of California, Anthem, and Aetna, now cover verification testing, particularly for the *BRCA* genes, Bonadies said. There are also research-grade testing options available through academic medical centers. Part of the challenge with this approach is that there are fewer than 5,000 genetic counselors in the United States who can provide the proper guidance based on these results (ABGC, 2019), and this challenge is likely to increase as gene panels become more complex and require more expert interpretation, Bonadies said.

Another avenue for integration could be through DTC medical-grade testing since there are now several laboratories offering this type of testing directly to consumers. On the other hand, some laboratories are pivoting away from a one-on-one interaction with a customer to large population-based studies, which could make it harder for consumers to access the services directly, Bonadies said.

An ongoing challenge will be getting back to patients with new information as research identifies more genetic associations with disease. "How do we reach back to our patients and notify them of those updates in the field?" Bonadies asked. Her group, for example, found that over the past 5 years there were more than 600 changes in medical management recommendations associated with the 59 genes that the American College of Medical Genetics and Genomics has identified as important for individuals to know if they have a pathogenic variant in those genes. "The medical system is not well set up to re-contact those patients and to keep them in the loop about their ever-evolving medical management and how they need to be followed," Bonadies said. The system that she and her colleagues have developed, however, does include the ability to reach out to patients and offer them the opportunity to participate in relevant clinical trials.

Bonadies proposed a vision of the future focusing on long-term engagement with consumers that offers verification programs, tools for health care providers, accessible and scalable genetic counseling, gene- and variant-specific reports, and updating reports with notifications that are important for medical management. Such a future would also include comprehensive, searchable resources for both patients and providers and focus on the engagement and retention of those patients and their providers.

LESSONS FROM A NEAR-CONSUMER TESTING EXPERIENCE

Describing the various types of genetic testing available today, Matthew Ferber discussed the spectrum ranging from purely diagnostic applications to what he called "edutainment"—how closely someone is related to Neanderthals, for example—and how the tests are ordered (i.e., via a provider or via more consumer-facing routes). DTC companies are now moving into the diagnostic space, he said, while the diagnostic companies are considering medically actionable mutations beyond *BRCA*.

Ferber said that when he first became a clinical laboratory director, he felt that genomics fell strictly in the medical sphere and that consumers might not understand the information received directly or that it might not be beneficial for them. Over the years, he said, his views have changed, and he now believes that DTC genomic testing creates an opportunity for people to talk about things that are important for their health, engage with their providers, and have meaningful conversations about genetics and genomics.

When the Mayo Clinic was deciding to launch its GeneGuide™ product, he said, one of the biggest concerns was not about the ability to interpret test results, but about keeping the cost of sequencing at a price affordable to the general consumer.[4] The breakthrough, Ferber said, came when Helix was able to provide low-cost, high-quality sequencing data with no interpretation. Combining Helix's expertise with the Mayo Clinic's expertise made for a good match, he added. The goal in creating a product like GeneGuide™ was to help people better understand genetics and genomics before they were faced with a critical result. It is not diagnostic testing, Ferber said, so people who suspect they may have hereditary breast or ovarian cancer in their family should not use this test. If an individual within the health system was determined to have an indication for clinical testing, Mayo's clinical partner, PWNHealth, would flag an individual's test order, and it would not go through the system. Instead, Ferber said, PWNHealth would help the individual find a genetic counselor in the area that he or she could work with to navigate next steps.

The result of this partnership was an entry-level product that sought to not overwhelm consumers yet at the same time provided an avenue for educating consumers and helping them understand how genetics can affect their health. The idea, Ferber said, is to use people's own genetic information to engage them in the process of learning about genetics. What he and his colleagues have learned, Ferber said, is that consumers enjoy learning about genomics but want more information about medically actionable variants, carrier screening, and pharmacogenomics information related to drugs they take.

An important difference between DTC tests and near-consumer tests, Ferber said, is that in the near-consumer environment consumers initiate the ordering process, but their physicians need to approve the orders and

---

[4]For more information about the Mayo Clinic GeneGuide™, see https://www.mayoclinic.org/mayoclinic-geneguide (accessed December 13, 2019).

receive copies of the results to review before they are sent to the consumers. Partnering with a health care provider can achieve the right balance, he added. This can be important in certain instances where there are additional factors at play, such as in the case of a consumer who has had a liver transplant, in which case the individual would metabolize medications like the liver donor and DTC results would not be accurate. In cases where consumers may receive critical results from a GeneGuide™ test (e.g., malignant hypothermia), the result would be held back for a genetic counselor to deliver. There have been many questions over the years about whether consumer-focused genomic testing should be done, Ferber said, but it is time to move past that conversation because such testing is here, and it is up to the field to try and figure out how to address related issues in the most appropriate manner.

DISCUSSION

Facilitators and Barriers to Integration

To start the discussion, panelists discussed impediments and facilitators of consumer genomics integration, ranging from including genomic sequencing results in electronic health records to the cost of and reimbursement for genomic sequencing. It is important, Singleton said, to consider the day in the near future when whole-genome sequencing will be inexpensive enough that everyone would be sequenced at birth and that information becomes part of their medical records. In his opinion, he said, this becomes a facilitator because it starts to turn health care systems into learning systems, where research and health care become one and the same. Ferber agreed that newborn screening with whole-genome sequencing could one day become routine, but added that DTC screening tests should not be done in otherwise healthy minors who do not have the ability to fully understand the gravity of an outcome or have complete say in what course of action to take based on an outcome.

Another facilitator, Dolan said, would be broadening the insurance coverage of genomics tests before receiving a diagnosis. Medicare, for example, does not pay for testing prior to diagnosis even when someone has a strong family history of cancer. "The opportunity to identify someone at risk and take steps is essentially precluded for many of my patients if Medicare will not pay because the out of pocket cost is too substantial," Dolan said. Another insurance-related facilitator would be to have a system where genetic counselors could be licensed and paid independently in every state, Dolan said, which would likely increase the supply of genetic counselors. One workshop participant referred to the challenges related to reimbursing pathologists and genetic counselors that had been discussed throughout the day and asked how Mayo developed its business plan for making its product available to patients. Activities like this are difficult in an academic medical setting, Ferber said, which is why partnerships have been crucial to the success of the GeneGuide™. In determining the price of the testing, Mayo negotiated with its partners based on the estimated number of people who might require additional genetic counseling, whether on the front end or following the test, and used that number to distribute costs. Insurance companies are not billed for the testing, which Ferber said helps spread costs. Reflecting on the comments in the session about partnerships, Blumberg added that one facilitator or barrier, depending on whether it is alignment or misalignment, could be how common the interests are between the various parties involved in the collaboration.

Overburdened clinicians asked to review and comment on a DTC genomics report are an impediment to integration, Bonadies said. Primary care physicians should not be expected to stay up to date with all of the various genetic conditions, she said. Along the same lines, Ferber said that the genomics field has not made it easy for clinicians to use the information they are getting now. In his opinion, he said, this issue could be addressed using clinical decision support tools integrated into the electronic health record. That said, getting data from DTC test services into the electronic health record will be a challenge and will require setting some standards to enable integration.

Data Quality and Data Sharing

One participant asked if there is a clear distinction between medical grade versus DTC genomic testing. Many DTC genomic tests are performed in Clinical Laboratory Improvement Amendments (CLIA)-approved laboratories, Bonadies replied, but she said that, as a genetic counselor, she would always repeat a DTC test in a medical grade laboratory to confirm a result. Drawing on her earlier presentation about variance between the data returned from the DTC genomic testing companies and medical grade laboratories, she said that the discrepancies occurred on both the level of variant interpretation and the interpretation of the raw sequencing data.

Research, clinical care, and drug development are likely going to intersect around DTC genomic tests, a workshop participant said, and it is not difficult to imagine needing to connect individuals with polygenic risk scores to clinical trials being done with pre-symptomatic patients in the future. There are current efforts to collect patients with *GBA* and *LRRK2* mutations for therapeutic development in the Parkinson's disease space, Singleton said, and the field is also moving toward engaging relatives who carry those mutations for clinical trials. Therapeutic development is still in its early days in this space, Singleton added, but there could be opportunities to better understand and interpret complex variant data. This could allow researchers to understand the genetic basis of diseases and to develop specific therapeutics for those individuals or even define subpopulations who could benefit from a therapeutic before becoming symptomatic. In terms of using polygenic risk scores, Singleton said, there is more caution because of the regulatory issues involved.

Moving from a paradigm in which the responsibility of re-contacting patients lies with the physician who ordered the test to a living lab report is a good concept, Ferber said. Communicating new information to patients about old genetic test results has always been challenging, Bonadies said. She described how as a genetic counselor she used to send a newsletter to patients that included a list of gene-related updates, which left patients to understand and determine which of those updates applied to them. My Gene Counsel has developed a living lab report, Bonadies added, which includes the ability to re-contact patients in order to connect them with new clinical trials as the knowledge about gene associations changes over time. The new living lab report model allows her company to connect with patients and their providers about specific genes and variants, which means that the patients do not have to sort through extra information that may not apply to them.

5

Regulatory and Health Policy Issues

Important Points Highlighted by Individual Speakers

- Several regulatory mechanisms, none comprehensive, exist to prevent access and restrict use of genetic data collected from consumers, though consumers may not be aware of these privacy protections. (Laser, McGuire)
- Law enforcement access to genomic data from direct-to-consumer (DTC) testing services is an issue that is receiving a lot of attention recently and may be of concern to consumers. (McGuire)
- The value of genetic research and benefits of genetic testing have to be weighed against potential privacy risks for consumers. (McGuire)
- It is not possible to completely protect privacy, so the goal should be to do the best job possible, make the regulations as transparent as possible, and engage the public in a way that increases trust. (McGuire)
- Reasons to regulate genomic testing services include to set metrics for analytical validity, clinical validity, and clinical utility; to set standards for the comprehensibility of the information provided to consumers and access to that information; and to protect and promote public health. (Javitt)
- Regulation of DTC genomic testing is complex and different components are overseen by various entities and agencies. As

the amount of genomic information available to physicians and patients continues to increase, it is increasingly important to develop consensus regarding the key objectives of regulation and the entities that are best placed to develop and implement policies to achieve these objectives. (Javitt)

- Best practices for DTC genomic test services focus on promoting transparency with respect to making sure that consumers get information in language they can understand, providing consumers with choices as far as whom they consent to have access to their data, enhancing privacy protections to include not sharing genetic data with employers and insurance companies, and requiring a legal process before disclosing data to law enforcement. (Laser)

The fourth workshop session, moderated by Victoria Pratt, the director of the Pharmacogenomics and Molecular Genetics Laboratories at the Indiana University School of Medicine, addressed data sharing, privacy, and security issues in the context of direct-to-consumer (DTC) genomics testing and explored the landscape of emerging regulatory issues in consumer genomics. Amy McGuire, the Leon Jaworski Professor of Biomedical Ethics and the director of the Center for Medical Ethics and Health Policy at the Baylor College of Medicine, focused her presentation on data sharing, privacy, and security. Gail Javitt, a member of the health care and life sciences practice at Epstein Becker Green, discussed the regulation of consumer genomics, and Jordan Laser, the senior director of cytogenetics and molecular pathology at the Long Island Jewish Medical Center and the chair of the professional relations committee of the Association for Molecular Pathology (AMP), spoke about AMP's position regarding the regulation of consumer genomics.

DATA SHARING, PRIVACY, AND SECURITY

Before ordering a DTC genomic test, McGuire said, consumers should review the company's privacy protections and understand who might have access to their data according to the accompanying terms of service. If a consumer genomics company violates its own terms of service, the consequences could include a citation by the Federal Trade Commission (FTC) for unlawful trade practices, fines, and potential lawsuits from consumers who suffered damages from that unlawful activity. However, McGuire said, violating the terms of service is not the only way in which consumers' information might be at risk and their privacy compromised, particularly when it comes to sharing genomic data.

McGuire discussed three groups that may legally obtain access to DTC genomic test data: researchers, those in the health care system, and various other actors such as members of law enforcement. There are a few ways to protect data privacy in the research and health care realms, McGuire said. The first is to protect against unauthorized access to protected data. One mechanism to do this relies on the Health Insurance Portability and Accountability Act (HIPAA). HIPAA protects against the unauthorized disclosure of protected health information by "covered entities," which includes health care systems. While companies that provide DTC genomics services may not themselves be covered entities, if the health care systems that receive data from them or directly from the consumer are covered entities, then they may not release the individual consumer's data without authorization, unless it is for the purpose of treatment, payment, or health care operations.

Certificates of confidentiality,[1] originally authorized by Congress in 1970, are a legal tool designed to protect the privacy of subjects in federally funded research that involves the collection of sensitive data. According to the 21st Century Cures Act, certificates of confidentiality must be issued by the Department of Health and Human Services to federally funded researchers who are collecting identifiable research data, and researchers who are not federally funded can apply for certificate protections (Wolf and Beskow, 2018). Certificates of confidentiality can protect against access by law enforcement and other actors even in the case of a subpoena or warrant, McGuire said. However, data that are not used for research are not protected by a certificate of confidentiality, she noted.

The second way to protect data privacy is to prevent the discriminatory use of those data. In 2008 Congress passed the Genetic Information Nondiscrimination Act (GINA), which prohibits health insurers and employers from using genetic information, including family health histories, for discriminatory purposes. GINA only applies to health insurers and companies with more than 50 employees; the law does not apply to life insurance, disability insurance, or long-term care policies. There has been heavy criticism of GINA for not being comprehensive in its protections, McGuire said. A national survey that McGuire and her collaborators conducted found that few people have ever heard of GINA, in contrast to HIPAA and the Americans with Disabilities Act (ADA). However, when her team explained what GINA was, 30 percent of the approximately 1,500 people surveyed said that they were less concerned about their privacy. The bad news, McGuire said, was that 30 percent of those surveyed felt more concerned about their privacy after learning about GINA because of the gaps in its protections.

---

[1]To read more about certificates of confidentiality and how they protect the privacy of research subjects in National Institutes of Health–funded research, see https://grants.nih.gov/policy/humansubjects/coc.htm (accessed December 9, 2019).

The Patient Protection and Affordable Care Act (ACA) and the ADA provide additional protections against genetic discrimination in the areas of health insurance and employment, McGuire said. Finally, she said, there are many states that have state-specific laws that provide even broader protections against genetic discrimination, with California having the most comprehensive state law.

Turning to the emerging issue of law enforcement access to consumer genomics information, McGuire shared the story of the search for a serial rapist, murderer, and armed robber who terrorized California between 1974 and 1986, known to law enforcement and in the media as the Golden State Killer. In 2018, after police had carried out more than 40 years of investigative work, Joseph DeAngelo was arrested and charged with eight counts of first degree murder and is accused of being the infamous Golden State Killer. During the course of their lengthy investigation, police tried to identify the Golden State Killer using numerous DNA samples obtained at the crime scenes, but were unsuccessful because his DNA was not in the national law enforcement database. Several years ago, a Federal Bureau of Investigation (FBI) agent decided to take a new approach, creating a variant profile from crime scene DNA samples and uploading it to a genetic genealogy database called GEDmatch. The database, McGuire explained, allows people to take their DTC genomic testing information and connect themselves with others in the database with whom they share DNA, suggesting a familial relation.

The aim of the FBI's approach was to identify relatives of the Golden State Killer, and, in fact, a third cousin was identified. The FBI then constructed a massive family tree using public databases, social media, and other sources, and focused on one individual who fit the profile: he was the right age, in the right places at the right time, and he was an ex-police officer. With a suspect in mind, law enforcement followed him and waited to collect DNA from his trash, and tests confirmed that Joseph DeAngelo's DNA was a match to the DNA collected at crime scenes linked to the Golden State Killer.

This approach has since been used in approximately 100 cases, McGuire said, with hundreds more in the pipeline. Some view this investigative tactic as an invasion of privacy and something that should not be permitted, McGuire said. Since the Golden State Killer case garnered widespread attention, companies have changed their terms of service to include language regarding law enforcement access to their customers' data. Ancestry.com and 23andMe, for example, will not provide access to their customers' information without a warrant, and GEDmatch now requires customers to opt into allowing law enforcement to access their information. As a result, the part of the GEDmatch database that is accessible to law enforcement went from 1.4 million people to about 180,000, which McGuire said significantly impedes law enforcement's ability to identify suspected criminals through familial matching. With regard to concerns about genetic privacy, McGuire said that law enforcement does not see a person's actual DNA sequence. Rather, they see what any other customer looking for a familial match would see—the name on the account for persons who share DNA with them, how much DNA they share, and the implications of that for how closely related they might be. One of the big questions in this space, McGuire said, is whether this violates the privacy of those individuals who match to the person who initiated the DTC testing.

Currently there are no regulations governing this type of use of genomic information, McGuire said. However, the field made strides recently in considering an appropriate path forward, with a Department of Justice interim policy that establishes parameters on the law enforcement use of non-forensic DNA databases for investigative purposes. This policy and other considerations were discussed at an October 2019 meeting that brought together state and federal law enforcement, company officials, consumer advocates, and other stakeholders.[2] In closing, McGuire said, there are always risks to privacy in today's world, and eliminating all risks in the area of consumer genetic testing is not possible. There are also counterbalancing values that are important to consider, such as the use of information to advance research, improve health, and protect public safety. At some point, trade-offs need to be made, McGuire said, and the conversation today is about how to make those trade-offs in a responsible and ethical manner.

REGULATION OF CONSUMER GENOMICS

There are three critical questions regarding the regulation of DTC genomic tests, Gail Javitt said: what to regulate, for what purposes regulations are needed, and who should do the regulating. There are many different aspects of consumer genomics that are currently or could be potentially regulated, including the laboratory performing the tests, the company selling test services, and marketing claims about the benefits of the products. Regulations could also specify the type of training and qualifications necessary to order a test and could govern the use of adjunctive products such as the software used to interpret the data, she said.

The reasons to regulate include setting standards for analytical validity, clinical validity, clinical utility, and the comprehensibility of the information provided to consumers; protecting access to that information; and, more broadly, protecting and promoting public health. For consumer genomics,

[2]The agenda for this meeting is available at https://www.cshl.edu/wp-content/uploads/2019/10/Privacy-Trust-Societal-Benefit-from-Consumer-Genomics-Meeting-Agenda-Banbury.pdf (accessed November 26, 2019).

Javitt said, the question of who should do the regulating is the toughest, most complicated, and most rapidly evolving part of the story. Federal agencies such as the Centers for Medicare & Medicaid Services (CMS), the Food and Drug Administration (FDA), and FTC are involved or potentially could be involved in the oversight of DTC genomic tests, she said, while states have primary authority over regulations pertaining to the health, safety, and welfare of their citizens, including the regulation of the health professions and the scope of laboratory and clinical practice. The courts also play a role in interpreting and enforcing regulations, and payers indirectly regulate the use of DTC genomic test services through their decisions on whether to pay for such tests. Finally, Javitt said, professional societies can establish professional norms that act as de facto regulations and oversight.

Each aspect of regulation of DTC genomic tests is fairly complex and can involve many different groups, Javitt said. For example, clinical laboratories that test samples for the purposes of health assessment are subject to the Clinical Laboratory Improvement Amendments (CLIA). CLIA regulates the quality of the facility, requires laboratories to hire people with certain types of training, and mandates documentation of analytical validity. Most states carry out the implementation and oversight of CLIA, Javitt said, although New York State is exempt from CLIA because its regulations are more rigorous. In the area of analytical validity, CMS has authorized the College of American Pathologists to perform laboratory certification in its stead. Laboratories also use a variety of instruments and tools that are regulated as medical devices by FDA under the Federal Food, Drug, and Cosmetic Act, she said.

One interesting aspect of regulation pertaining to DTC genomic tests has to do with laboratory-developed tests (LDTs), which are tests that laboratories develop for their own internal use instead of using a commercially available, FDA-approved kit. While FDA has the authority to regulate LDTs, it has largely decided to exercise its "enforcement discretion" (meaning to not take enforcement action), Javitt said, although FDA has, in limited circumstances, sent warning letters to specific laboratories objecting to specific LDTs. The FTC is responsible for regulating advertising and promotional claims under its authority to prohibit unfair trade practices, including the use of deceptive advertising. For the most part, the FTC has not initiated actions against DTC genomics companies for their marketing claims, Javitt said (although they have in a few circumstances investigated the privacy practices of certain DTC companies). The FTC also maintains a website with relevant information for consumers who are considering this type of test.[3]

[3]The FTC provides information to consumers on DTC genetic tests at https://www.consumer.ftc.gov/articles/0166-direct-consumer-genetic-tests (accessed December 10, 2019).

Javitt said that for many years FDA has sent mixed signals regarding its regulatory intentions with respect to LDTs. For example, in 2006 and 2007 FDA released draft guidance for the regulation of in vitro diagnostic multivariate index assays, which are tests that use proprietary algorithms to analyze multiple biomarkers and generate a risk score; however, the guidance was never finalized, and FDA did not end up regulating those assays. Subsequently, in 2010 FDA announced it would regulate DTC genomic tests and companies and that all DTC genomic tests that provided health information in the absence of FDA review were unlawful. As a result, Javitt said, a number of companies changed their business models. In 2013 FDA sent warning letters to five companies, including 23andMe, Navigenics, and DeCode, letting them know that their genetic test offerings were considered a medical device and had not received proper regulatory clearance. At that point, 23andMe stopped offering health-related information and began submitting a number of applications for its tests to FDA, some of which have been authorized for marketing and are once again offered to customers. In 2016, FDA announced that it would not be finalizing a framework for LDT oversight in order to allow for additional public discussion and for Congress to develop a legislative solution. More recently, however, FDA has taken steps to prohibit laboratories from offering pharmacogenomics tests on the basis that, in the agency's view, the relationship between DNA variations and medication response has not been established (see Table 5-1).

TABLE 5-1 Recent Developments Regarding the Regulation of Pharmacogenomics Tests (as presented by Gail Javitt on October 29, 2019)

Date	Action	Summary
October 31, 2018	The Food and Drug Administration (FDA) issues safety communication warning[a] against the use of pharmacogenomics tests	• Warning to health care providers that the link between DNA variants and the effect of most medications has not yet been established. • Health care providers should gather information from FDA-approved drug labels about whether genetic information should be used for determining therapeutic treatment. • Warning to patients that most genetic tests that make claims about the effects of a specific medicine are not supported by enough scientific or clinical evidence. • Recommends that test developers and manufacturers assure that the test report and product labeling support an intended use that aligns with the FDA-approved use of the medication.

continued

TABLE 5-1 Continued

Date	Action	Summary
April 4, 2019	FDA issues a warning letter[b] to Inova Genomics Laboratory	• Alleges that the MediMap genetic tests lack evidence of clinical validity and may affect health care providers' decision making in ways that are detrimental to patient health.
Summer 2019	FDA contacts various entities offering pharmacogenomics testing	• FDA reached out to several firms marketing pharmacogenetic tests that claim to predict how a person will respond to specific medications in instances where the association between the genetic variants and the medication's effects have not yet been established. • Most firms addressed FDA's concerns by removing specific medication names from their labeling, including promotional material and patient test reports.
September 2019	American Clinical Laboratory Association (ACLA) submits a letter to FDA Association for Molecular Pathology (AMP) issues a statement on "best practices" for pharmacogenomics testing	• ACLA letter: Concern that FDA's action will result in the loss of actionable information that providers rely on to make informed prescribing decisions. • AMP Statement: Encourages the use of Clinical Pharmacogenetics Implementation Consortium gene–drug practice guidelines and states that clinically meaningful pharmacogenetic test results can improve patient care and professional practice (under certain conditions).

[a]The full text from the FDA safety communication warning regarding the use of genetic tests with unapproved claims to predict patient response to medications from October 2018 is available at https://www.fda.gov/medical-devices/safety-communications/fda-warns-against-use-many-genetic-tests-unapproved-claims-predict-patient-response-specific (accessed December 10, 2019).

[b]The warning letter from FDA to the Inova Genomics Laboratory can be found at https://www.fda.gov/inspections-compliance-enforcement-and-criminal-investigations/warning-letters/inova-genomics-laboratory-577422-04042019 (accessed December 10, 2019).

The regulation of DTC genomic testing is not simple or straightforward, Javitt said. The delivery of DTC genomic testing includes a number of different activities that are or could be regulated, she said, and different regulatory bodies are responsible, or potentially responsible, for these activities. Who has jurisdiction over some activities remains unclear, and there has been a lack of a coherent or consistent regulatory framework for other activities. "As the amount of genomic information available continues to increase,"

Javitt said, "it is increasingly important to develop consensus regarding the key objectives of regulation and the entities that are best placed to develop and implement policies to achieve these objectives."

THE ASSOCIATION FOR MOLECULAR PATHOLOGY'S EVOLVING POSITION ON CONSUMER GENOMICS

Jordan Laser used the evolving position statement of AMP as an example to illustrate how the field of consumer genomics testing is changing and some of the current concerns about regulation and privacy. AMP's first position statement, issued in 2007, reflected the concern that consumers who ordered such tests directly would not be able to fully understand the test results. "Back then we only felt comfortable with such tests being ordered and interpreted through the context of a health care provider," Laser said. AMP also felt strongly that genomic tests should only be conducted in a laboratory regulated by CLIA.

With the evolution and massive growth of the DTC genomic test industry, AMP changed its position statement in 2015. The group recognized that DTC testing was likely here to stay and that it could provide some level of value, Laser said, so the position statement was updated to support DTC testing with some conditions. AMP remained neutral regarding ancestry testing, deciding that such information posed little risk to the consumer and might lead to an increase in genetic literacy among the public. The group did oppose consumer genetic testing for which the company would then offer secondary services, such as vitamins, movies, and books, that were targeted to specific individuals, he said.

In 2019 AMP updated its position statement once again to reflect another stage in the field's evolution. The 2019 statement[4] delved more deeply and broadly into the issue of transparency around consumers' ability to understand their results in terms of analytical and clinical validity. The statement also covered the need to educate consumers about the uses and limitations of these tests, and it recommended referrals to genetic counselors to support consumers. The most important addition to the 2019 position statement, Laser said, was a discussion on privacy protections and on the Future of Privacy Forum's work[5] on developing privacy best practices for consumer genomic testing services. These best practices focus on promoting transparency with respect to making sure that consumers get

[4]The 2019 AMP position statement is available at https://www.amp.org/AMP/assets/File/position-statements/2019/AMP_Position_Statement_Consumer_Genomics_FINAL.pdf?pass=63 (accessed November 26, 2019).

[5]The Future of Privacy Forum's document titled Privacy Best Practices for Consumer Genetic Testing Services is available at https://fpf.org/wp-content/uploads/2018/07/Privacy-Best-Practices-for-Consumer-Genetic-Testing-Services-FINAL.pdf (accessed December 11, 2019).

information in language they can understand, providing consumers with choices concerning who has permission to access their data, enhancing privacy protections to include not sharing genetic data with employers and insurance companies, and requiring a legal process before disclosing data to law enforcement.

Laser pointed out several areas where privacy and regulatory protections related to DTC genomic testing have been instituted. The ADA, for example, includes a provision that prevents employment discrimination based on genetic information, Laser noted, and the ACA's provisions on preexisting conditions includes genetic information. The Code of Federal Regulations, Title 45 Part 46, also provides a number of protections for data used in research.[6] The issue is not so much that there are no regulations concerning privacy protections, Laser said, but rather that most consumers do not know about them.

States also offer legal and regulatory protections for consumers, including protection against genetic discrimination by insurers and employers. Several states have also added their own provisions to strengthen GINA by instituting nondiscrimination protections regarding life, disability, and long-term care insurance. For example, Laser said, California has its own expanded version of GINA that also covers emergency medical services, housing, mortgage lending, education, and other state-funded programs.

DISCUSSION

Regulatory Gaps for Direct-to-Consumer Genomic Tests

Vicky Pratt asked where the regulatory and privacy gaps for consumer genomics are. Currently, Laser said, there is a patchwork of protections in place rather than one comprehensive level of protection, and there are concerns that consumers are not aware of these protections and may not know how to navigate them. It is going to be very difficult to build guardrails that completely protect privacy in the DTC genomics space, McGuire added. The goals should be to do the best job possible, to make the regulations as transparent as possible, and to engage the public in a way that increases trust, McGuire said. Another important issue to consider, Javitt said, is the increasing convergence of DTC genomics companies and health care delivery systems. It may be more challenging to try to consider regulatory issues in those two spheres separately because many of the concerns are the same, regardless of who is ordering the test and seeing the results first. An

[6]For more information on the protection of human research subjects, see https://www.govinfo.gov/content/pkg/CFR-2016-title45-vol1/pdf/CFR-2016-title45-vol1-part46.pdf (accessed January 10, 2020).

important step in moving forward with the regulation of DTC genomics, Javitt said, will be gaining consensus concerning what the appropriate risk tolerance should be regarding the validation of evidence. Since that could be a messy and time-consuming process, she said, in the interim consumers should try to be aware of the limitations of the tests they are taking, and companies should try to not oversell their products.

Many consumers may not be aware of third-party companies that offer to interpret the raw data from DTC genomic tests, Pomerantz said, and she asked the panelists how those companies are regulated and by whom. Companies that interpret raw DTC genomic data but do not actually perform the sequencing (sometimes referred to as dry laboratories) represent an area that is falling through the regulatory cracks, Javitt said. In New York State, she said, these companies would likely meet the definition of a laboratory and be subject to that state's Clinical Laboratory Evaluation Program.[7] It is not clear, though, if there is enforcement action, she said. The other potential area of oversight for third-party interpretation companies involves their proprietary software, Javitt said. It is unclear if that software is subject to FDA regulation as medical devices, she said, and although it is very important, this area is not receiving a lot of attention at the moment.

A workshop participant suggested that consumers should have an ongoing ability to request that their data be deleted. The participant also said that consumers should be informed as to whether there is foreign involvement in the companies that offer these tests, a point with which Laser agreed.

Privacy and Genetic Exceptionalism

One workshop participant asked whether there was a need for specific language and federal privacy legislation concerning genomic data. The debate about providing a higher level of privacy protection for genomic information has been going on for a long time, McGuire said, and there are good arguments on both sides. The recent familial matching by law enforcement raises distinctive issues that do require more thought, she added. Balancing privacy, innovation, and research has always been a challenge, Laser said. A world of absolute privacy does not really allow for innovation and effective research, he said, and genetic exceptionalism may be the result of our current level of discomfort around the available evidence. Over time, he said, as more data are collected, one hopes that the discomfort concerning genetics will subside.

---

[7]More information on the New York State Clinical Laboratory Evaluation Program can be found at https://www.wadsworth.org/regulatory/clep (accessed on December 12, 2019).

Possible Role for Direct-to-Consumer Genomics Companies in Cascade Screening

DTC genomic tests can sometimes have a big impact on families, Geoff Ginsburg said. Cascade screening, the process of contacting family members who may be at risk for a pathogenic variant, is currently quite challenging within the context of the American health care system, in part because of HIPAA regulations, he continued. Perhaps cascade screening would be more effective and easier if it were conducted through the DTC genomics companies instead of within the health care system, because the companies are often not considered covered entities under HIPAA and therefore have more freedom. Many companies may still have confidentiality and privacy rules laid out in their terms and conditions, McGuire said, so any contact of family members would have to abide by those rules. The FTC can also investigate DTC genomics companies for privacy violations, Javitt said, so companies must ensure that the activities they conduct are in line with their stated privacy policies.

6

How Can Consumer Genomics Be Better Integrated to Improve Health?

Important Points Highlighted by Individual Speakers

- Research is needed to better understand what a particular genetic change means, how to annotate it, and how to interpret those variations. (Stenzel)
- Direct-to-consumer (DTC) genomic services could provide more directive resources to consumers to help them determine the next steps they might take, given their family histories and the results of their tests. (Bonadies)
- Offering pretest counseling, or at least a checklist for consumers outlining the limitations of certain testing and the appropriateness for them, could be a way to resolve some of the tension between larger genetic testing panels and genetic tests customized for the individual. (Dolan, Nussbaum)
- Hybrid models could be a solution for bringing clinicians into the consumer genomics process. (Nussbaum)
- Companies should be incentivized to share their data, particularly for underrepresented populations, and deposit them in publicly accessible databases. (Callier, Nussbaum)
- The volume of data generated by consumer genomics companies could create incentives for electronic health record companies to develop standards for interoperability and maintenance of genomic data in the context of health care systems. (Feero)

- Fund research that would use computer algorithms and artificial intelligence to create automated systems that would perform some of the interpretation functions and help ameliorate the shortage of genetic counselors. (Ferber)
- Research is needed to determine which consumers will benefit the most from having genetic counseling services and how best to "tier" those individuals to allow genetic counselors to practice more efficiently. (Wicklund)
- Consider an implementation science approach for defining the challenges (e.g., consumer and provider education) and other aspects of integrating consumer genomics into clinical practice. (Wicklund)

INTEGRATING CONSUMER GENOMICS INTO THE HEALTH SYSTEM

Hunt Willard, the director of Geisinger National Precision Health and the session's moderator said that this had been one of the first meetings in which he had seen recognition of the fact that the health care ecosystem has changed substantially to the point that it is now organized around health systems rather than individual provider practices. Gone are the days in which a single doctor would take care of a patient and all of that person's health care went through either a local primary care physician or a local hospital, Willard continued. There are individual hospitals, but now consumers are more likely not entering the health care ecosystem through a clinical provider or a clinic. That relationship between people and their providers has changed, he said; many people may not know who their health system is, but they know the clinic they go to and their usual provider, even if that provider actually may change every time they go to that clinic. A health system point of reference may be important only if someone has a reason to visit a hospital for a medical event.

Many people may only engage with the health ecosystem when they want or need it. They may even pick and choose how to interact with certain parts of the ecosystem, Willard said. That may be the future of how people use the health care system and ecosystem.

Reflections on Consumer Genomics in the Health System

The workshop's final session was a panel discussion in which the panelists were asked to reflect on what they had heard during the day's previous sessions. In particular, the panelists were asked to explore what the role of consumer genomics might be in the health care system over the next 5 to 10 years and whether health systems, consumers, and providers are prepared for the downstream challenges that will arise as consumer genomics finds more effective uses in clinical care. The panelists who participated in this part of the day were Danielle Bonadies, Shawneequa Callier, Siobhan Dolan, Robert Nussbaum, Dorothy Pomerantz, and Timothy Stenzel, the director of the Office of In Vitro Diagnostics and Radiological Health in the Office of Product Evaluation and Quality at the Food and Drug Administration's (FDA's) Center for Devices and Radiological Health.

Stenzel noted that in the case of consumer genetics and genomics, before granting approval for a specific test or system, FDA examines its analytical and clinical validity, whether it is safe and effective, and its benefits and risks.[1] For example, in the case of a direct-to-consumer (DTC) genomic test the agency was aware that a physician may not be involved in receiving and interpreting the results of the test, so it was important for FDA to see the results of usability studies before it granted approval. Stenzel, speaking about what he found to be the most important messages of the day, cited the importance of getting more consumer and patient input into this field as it moves forward. In particular, he said that he had heard during the workshop that in many ways the system works as it should—it is safe—and that there may be ways to enhance the system so that when consumers receive a concerning test result, they will have more support to deal with that result.

Nussbaum said his major takeaway from the day was that the system is not at equilibrium because of contradictions that were exposed during the day:

- People have a greater thirst for genetic information than is being satisfied by the traditional medical system;
- There are logistical barriers to people being able to acquire that information;
- If consumers ignore the medical establishment by ordering a test directly from a DTC service and they have a strongly positive test of some sort, they want the medical establishment involved again. There is not enough person power in the medical system to be able to provide that type of support; and
- People want an inexpensive test, but at the same time someone has to pay the genetic counselor for the time and effort spent caring for a patient when there is a strongly positive result.

---

[1]Lists of DTC tests with marketing authorization: https://www.fda.gov/medical-devices/vitro-diagnostics/direct-consumer-tests#list (accessed December 10, 2019).

These challenges are complex, Nussbaum said. "The solution to this problem is going to require a multifactorial approach that attacks many of those inconsistencies and contradictions," he added.

Dolan said that she was struck by the issues of access and navigation, how they vary by health care system, and how they affect a person's sense of empowerment. For example, when she sees a patient who has a mutation associated with an increased risk of cancer, she tells the patient that part of the experience is for her to help change the patient's view of the information from feeling that it is something troubling to something that is empowering. "I have always had the sense," she said, "that it is critically important to find a way to assist the patient to make that transition and use this genetic information to be empowering." Dolan also highlighted the transparency issues related to the cost of testing and follow-up care. Consumer genomics is more straightforward in terms of the payment for the service that the consumer receives than is clinical care delivery, which can be less transparent. But if a way is not found to engage diverse populations and provide less expensive testing options, she said, the result could be an increase in disparities.

Callier said an issue she was grappling with after the day's discussions was where the line is drawn between the medical system and the consumer environment regarding regulations and data protections, particularly for data access by law enforcement. She voiced concern that law enforcement's use of genetic databases could discourage individuals from underrepresented populations from participating in genomics research.

Bonadies said that the field is not fulfilling its obligation in terms of identifying those who may be at increased risk of certain genetic conditions. The Centers for Disease Control and Prevention (CDC) has identified three genomic conditions it considers important for health care providers to identify and diagnose in individuals—hereditary breast and ovarian cancer syndrome, Lynch syndrome, and familial hypercholesterolemia.[2] Despite this, only 30 percent of women diagnosed with ovarian cancer have been tested for associated mutations, she said. It is her hope that DTC genomic testing can narrow that gap and help build bridges to the medical system, but that will require tools that consumers can use to determine which test might be best for them, given their family histories and other factors.

One way to address this, Bonadies added, could be for DTC genomic services to provide more directive resources to consumers that would help them determine the next steps they might take, given their family histories

[2]For more information about the CDC Tier 1 genomic applications, see https://www.cdc.gov/genomics/implementation/toolkit/tier1.htm (accessed January 28, 2020). Note: Murray et al. (2018) have suggested that these Tier 1 conditions could be implemented in a genomics-based screening program.

and the results of their tests. This kind of tool would put more responsibility in the hands of DTC services and not add a burden to primary care physicians or disrupt their workflow, Willard said, adding that any plan that would add such burdens to physicians would be a nonstarter. Bonadies also said that the University of California, San Francisco, now has a clinic dedicated to working with people who have had DTC genomics tests and getting those individuals connected into primary care as well as providing confirmatory tests.

Dolan suggested creating more possibilities for pretest counseling as a means of both forming relationships with potential patients and also directing them to the appropriate tests and away from tests that would have no value. For example, at one point her clinic was seeing women of Puerto Rican and Dominican ancestry who were coming in with results of an Ashkenazi Jewish *BRCA* carrier screening panel, which was completely inappropriate. In her view, she said, there is a tension between the development of bigger and better panels of markers and customizing tests for specific individuals; offering pretest counseling, or at least a checklist for consumers, is the way to resolve that tension, she said. Nussbaum suggested thinking about pretest counseling as a form of triage.

Ferber predicted that DTC testing and physician-ordered testing are going to merge as the technologies continue to evolve. That may be, Michelle Penny said, but providing results to the individual in a fit-for-purpose manner and interpreting those results will still be a limiting factor in how valuable these tests will be, whether the consumer is using them to explore ancestry or to explore possible health issues. Asking physicians to add these interpretations to their workflows means that something else will need to be given up so as to not overburden them, she said. Penny then asked the panelists for their ideas about making more use of patient advocacy groups and registries, as The Michael J. Fox Foundation for Parkinson's Research is doing, to connect DTC services and health care. Dolan strongly supported that idea, saying that there is a wealth of expertise within those communities that could be tapped.

Advancing the Research

Geoffrey Ginsburg asked the panelists for their ideas on the most compelling research questions that the National Human Genome Research Institute (NHGRI) should consider funding to advance the field. Nussbaum said that a concerted effort is needed to achieve a level of information about genotype and phenotype correlations for people with ancestry other than from northern Europe that is comparable to the information available to those with European ancestry, and Callier called for an effort to incentivize companies to share their data, particularly for underrepresented populations, and deposit those data in publicly accessible databases. Nussbaum responded that one incentive would be that if companies do not put data into the federal ClinVar database, which aggregates information about genomic variation and its relationship to human health,[3] their tests would not receive Clinical Laboratory Improvement Amendments certification, and they would not be reimbursed by the Centers for Medicare & Medicaid Services or other payers. He said that ClinVar is an important quality control tool because it allows for cross-comparison of variant interpretation across laboratories.

Stenzel suggested funding research to understand what a particular genetic change means, how to annotate it, and how to interpret the variations. Ferber proposed funding research that would use computer algorithms and artificial intelligence to create automated systems that would perform some of the interpretation functions and help ameliorate some of the workforce issues discussed throughout the day. Along those lines, Wicklund said that research could help answer the question of who can best benefit from seeing a genetic counselor, and Bonadies noted that her team is providing baseline education along with test results so that when people do go see a genetic counselor, they can then drill down on specific questions related to their family history and risk in order to use the appointment time more efficiently. One workshop participant noted that NHGRI once led the Genomic Literacy, Education, and Engagement Initiative which put a great deal of thought into how to educate students, providers, and consumers. Unfortunately, she said, this effort did not receive enough funding to move forward, but there could be an opportunity for the field to come together to focus those resources in a more centralized manner and avoid duplicative efforts.

CONCLUDING REMARKS

Greg Feero and Cathy Wicklund concluded the workshop with a few summary remarks and potential next steps that the roundtable and the genomics community could explore (see Box 6-1). Feero commented that nearly every speaker had made it abundantly clear that there is a need to increase the amount of data from underrepresented populations in genomics databases if the benefits of genomic testing, whether via the DTC or clinical route, are to extend to all segments of the population, not just those of European ancestry.

Feero then highlighted the need to consider how to facilitate the use, upkeep, and secure storage of genomic information over time and what

[3]For more information on ClinVar, see https://www.ncbi.nlm.nih.gov/clinvar (accessed January 10, 2020).

BOX 6-1
Potential Next Steps for the Roundtable and the Genomics Community (as presented by Greg Feero)

- Explore approaches to incentivize the collection of more data from underserved populations and the deposition of those data into publicly accessible databases, including data collected by direct-to-consumer (DTC) genomic services. This could include convening stakeholders and helping to leverage partnerships to create a more diverse evidence base.
- Examine ways of facilitating connections between community groups and educational resources for DTC testing.
- Consider approaches for developing systems to support providers and patients in the event that DTC testing returns an actionable result as a means of reducing the gap between obtaining DTC results and engaging with the health care system.
- Discuss approaches for incorporating risk algorithms and explaining error bars when returning results to consumers.
- Explore whether the large DTC-adopting population, expected to reach 100 million consumers in the near future, is incentive enough for electronic health record vendors to develop approaches for integrating consumer genomics data into the electronic health record.
- Convene stakeholders more deliberately to discuss the impact of DTC genomic tests on the health care system.
- Explore facilitating the establishment of partnerships between DTC genomic services and the pharmaceutical industry to improve drug development efforts.

the roles of the various actors in the field should be in that regard. Doing so was challenging before DTC testing became available, he said, and advances in that realm have added a new wrinkle to this challenge. There is a need for increased transparency so that all patients and providers can understand the benefits and limitations of data and around data security and sharing policies for both patients and providers, he said. Increased clarity concerning regulations in the genomic testing space will be important for both DTC and clinical tests, as will be increased transparency regarding the protections for consumers related to discrimination and how consumers' information will be used.

In closing, Feero highlighted the importance of better understanding who is using DTC genomic services, what their attitudes and interests are regarding these tests and the information they can provide, and what their views are on secondary uses of their information and how that information is integrated into clinical care. At this point, he said, such information comes mostly from early adopters, and he suspects it would be interesting to compare the motivations of the early adopters to those who are coming into the system today. Wicklund added that such information would also indicate whether genomic tests are penetrating into underserved populations and perhaps provide insights into how to increase uptake by those populations.

Final Thoughts

Pomeranz told the workshop audience that she wished that everybody who ever had a genetic test could have the opportunity to participate in a similar roundtable workshop. The challenges with educating consumers are part of the process with a technology this new, she added, but there is a real need for more education. "Because we are engaging directly with these at-home genetic testing companies and asking them to tell us really important things about our genetics," she said, "I wish that we had better education and we knew more." The number of individuals who have been introduced to the idea of genetics through DTC testing is substantial, Bonadies said, adding that this is a great opportunity for the field to build bridges back to the traditional medical system and use those data to confirm results and improve overall health.

References

ABGC (American Board of Genetic Counseling). 2019. *Mission statement, purpose and values.* https://www.abgc.net/about-abgc/mission-history (accessed December 13, 2019).

Allyse, M. A., D. H. Robinson, M. J. Ferber, and R. R. Sharp. 2018. Direct-to-consumer testing 2.0: Emerging models of direct-to-consumer genetic testing. *Mayo Clinic Proceedings* 93(1):113–120.

Auer, P. L., A. P. Reiner, G. Wang, H. M. Kang, G. R. Abecasis, D. Altshuler, M. J. Bamshad, D. A. Nickerson, R. P. Tracy, S. S. Rich, and S. M. Leal. 2016. Guidelines for large-scale sequence-based complex trait association studies: Lessons learned from the NHLBI exome sequencing project. *American Journal of Human Genetics* 99(4):791–801.

Blell, M., and M. A. Hunter. 2019. Direct-to-consumer genetic testing's red herring: "Genetic ancestry" and personalized medicine. *Frontiers in Medicine* 6:48.

Bloss, C. S., L. Ornowski, E. Silver, M. Cargill, V. Vanier, N. J. Schork, and E. J. Topol. 2010. Consumer perceptions of direct-to-consumer personalized genomic risk assessments. *Genetics in Medicine* 12(9):556–566.

Bonham, V. L., E. D. Green, and E. J. Pérez-Stable. 2018. Examining how race, ethnicity, and ancestry data are used in biomedical research. *JAMA* 320(15):1533–1534.

Brasler, K. 2019. *DNA ancestry testing: Are their reports rooted in reality?* https://www.checkbook.org/national/dna-ancestry-services/articles/DNA-Ancestry-Testing-Are-Their-Reports-Rooted-in-Reality-7242 (accessed November 22, 2019).

Caswell-Jin, J. L., T. Gupta, E. Hall, I. M. Petrovchich, M. A. Mills, K. E. Kingham, R. Koff, N. M. Chun, P. Levonian, A. P. Lebensohn, J. M. Ford, and A. W. Kurian. 2018. Racial/ethnic differences in multiple-gene sequencing results for hereditary cancer risk. *Genetics in Medicine* 20(2):234–239.

Cooper, R. S., G. N. Nadkarni, and G. Ogedegbe. 2018. Race, ancestry, and reporting in medical journals. *JAMA* 320(15):1531–1532.

Darst, B. F., L. Madlensky, N. J. Schork, E. J. Topol, and C. S. Bloss. 2014. Characteristics of genomic test consumers who spontaneously share results with their health care provider. *Health Communication* 29(1):105–108.

Do, C. B., J. Y. Tung, E. Dorfman, A. K. Kiefer, E. M. Drabant, U. Francke, J. L. Mountain, S. M. Goldman, C. M. Tanner, J. W. Langston, A. Wojcicki, and N. Eriksson. 2011. Web-based genome-wide association study identifies two novel loci and a substantial genetic component for parkinson's disease. *PLOS Genetics* 7(6):e1002141.

Fogleman, A. J., W. E. Zahnd, A. E. Lipka, R. S. Malhi, S. Ganai, K. R. Delfino, and W. D. Jenkins. 2019. Knowledge, attitudes, and perceived barriers towards genetic testing across three rural Illinois communities. *Journal of Community Genetics* 10(3):417–423.

Goldsmith, L., L. Jackson, A. O'Connor, and H. Skirton. 2012. Direct-to-consumer genomic testing: Systematic review of the literature on user perspectives. *European Journal of Human Genetics* 20(8):811–816.

Gray, S. W., S. E. Gollust, D. A. Carere, C. A. Chen, A. Cronin, S. S. Kalia, H. Q. Rana, M. T. Ruffin IV, C. Wang, J. S. Roberts, and R. C. Green. 2017. Personal genomic testing for cancer risk: Results from the Impact of Personal Genomics study. *Journal of Clinical Oncology* 35(6):636–644.

Hollands, G. J., S. C. Whitwell, R. A. Parker, N. J. Prescott, A. Forbes, J. Sanderson, C. G. Mathew, C. M. Lewis, S. Watts, S. Sutton, D. Armstrong, A. L. Kinmonth, A. T. Prevost, and T. M. Marteau. 2012. Effect of communicating DNA based risk assessments for Crohn's disease on smoking cessation: Randomised controlled trial. *British Medical Journal* 345:e4708.

Hollands, G. J., D. P. French, S. J. Griffin, A. T. Prevost, S. Sutton, S. King, and T. M. Marteau. 2016. The impact of communicating genetic risks of disease on risk-reducing health behaviour: Systematic review with meta-analysis. *British Medical Journal* 352:i1102.

Howlader, N., A.M. Noone, M. Krapcho, D. Miller, A. Brest, M. Yu, J. Ruhl, Z. Tatalovich, A. Mariotto, D. R. Lewis, H. S. Chen, E. J. Feuer, and K. A. Cronin (Eds.). 2019. *SEER cancer statistics review, 1975–2016*. National Cancer Institute. Bethesda, MD. Based on November 2018 SEER data submission, posted to the SEER website, April 2019. https://seer.cancer.gov/csr/1975_2016 (accessed January 20, 2020).

IPDGC and WTCCC2 (International Parkinson Disease Genomics Consortium and Wellcome Trust Case Control Consortium 2). 2011. A two-stage meta-analysis identifies several new loci for Parkinson's disease. *PLOS Genetics* 7(6):e1002142.

Kaphingst, K. A., C. M. McBride, C. Wade, S. H. Alford, R. Reid, E. Larson, A. D. Baxevanis, and L. C. Brody. 2012. Patients' understanding of and responses to multiplex genetic susceptibility test results. *Genetics in Medicine* 14(7):681–687.

Khan, R., and D. Mittelman. 2018. Consumer genomics will change your life, whether you get tested or not. *Genome Biology* 19(1):120.

Khoury, M. J., C. M. McBride, S. D. Schully, J. P. Ioannidis, W. G. Feero, A. C. Janssens, M. Gwinn, D. G. Simons-Morton, J. M. Bernhardt, M. Cargill, S. J. Chanock, G. M. Church, R. J. Coates, F. S. Collins, R. T. Croyle, B. R. Davis, G. J. Downing, A. Duross, S. Friedman, M. H. Gail, G. S. Ginsburg, R. C. Green, M. H. Greene, P. Greenland, J. R. Gulcher, A. Hsu, K. L. Hudson, S. L. Kardia, P. L. Kimmel, M. S. Lauer, A. M. Miller, K. Offit, D. F. Ransohoff, J. S. Roberts, R. S. Rasooly, K. Stefansson, S. F. Terry, S. M. Teutsch, A. Trepanier, K. L. Wanke, J. S. Witte, and J. Xu. 2009. The scientific foundation for personal genomics: Recommendations from a National Institutes of Health–Centers for Disease Control and Prevention multidisciplinary workshop. *Genetics in Medicine* 11(8):559–567.

Krieger, J. L., F. Murray, J. S. Roberts, and R. C. Green. 2016. The impact of personal genomics on risk perceptions and medical decision-making. *Nature Biotechnology* 34(9):912–918.

Kuchenbaecker, K. B., J. L. Hopper, D. R. Barnes, K. A. Phillips, T. M. Mooij, M. J. Roos-Blom, S. Jervis, F. E. van Leeuwen, R. L. Milne, N. Andrieu, D. E. Goldgar, M. B. Terry, M. A. Rookus, D. F. Easton, A. C. Antoniou, L. McGuffog, D. G. Evans, D. Barrowdale, D. Frost, J. Adlard, K. R. Ong, L. Izatt, M. Tischkowitz, R. Eeles, R. Davidson, S. Hodgson, S. Ellis, C. Nogues, C. Lasset, D. Stoppa-Lyonnet, J. P. Fricker, L. Faivre, P. Berthet, M. J. Hooning, L. E. van der Kolk, C. M. Kets, M. A. Adank, E. M. John, W. K. Chung, I. L. Andrulis, M. Southey, M. B. Daly, S. S. Buys, A. Osorio, C. Engel, K. Kast, R. K. Schmutzler, T. Caldes, A. Jakubowska, J. Simard, M. L. Friedlander, S. A. McLachlan, E. Machackova, L. Foretova, Y. Y. Tan, C. F. Singer, E. Olah, A. M. Gerdes, B. Arver, and H. Olsson. 2017. Risks of breast, ovarian, and contralateral breast cancer for BRCA1 and BRCA2 mutation carriers. *JAMA* 317(23):2402–2416.

Landry, L., D. E. Nielsen, D. A. Carere, J. S. Roberts, R. C. Green, and P. G. S. Group. 2017. Racial minority group interest in direct-to-consumer genetic testing: Findings from the PGen study. *Journal of Community Genetics* 8(4):293–301.

Landry, L. G., N. Ali, D. R. Williams, H. L. Rehm, and V. L. Bonham. 2018. Lack of diversity in genomic databases is a barrier to translating precision medicine research into practice. *Health Affairs (Millwood)* 37(5):780–785.

Mallow, J. A., L. A. Theeke, P. Crawford, E. Prendergast, C. Conner, T. Richards, B. McKown, D. Bush, D. Reed, M. E. Stabler, J. Zhang, G. Dino, and T. L. Barr. 2016. Understanding genomic knowledge in rural Appalachia: The West Virginia Genome Community Project. *Online Journal of Rural Nursing and Health Care* 16(1):3–22.

Manrai, A. K., B. H. Funke, H. L. Rehm, M. S. Olesen, B. A. Maron, P. Szolovits, D. M. Margulies, J. Loscalzo, and I. S. Kohane. 2016. Genetic misdiagnoses and the potential for health disparities. *New England Journal of Medicine* 375(7):655–665.

Martin, A. R., M. Kanai, Y. Kamatani, Y. Okada, B. M. Neale, and M. J. Daly. 2019. Clinical use of current polygenic risk scores may exacerbate health disparities. *Nature Genetics* 51(4):584–591.

Murray, M. F., J. P. Evans, M. Angrist, K. Chan, W. Uhlmann, D. L. Doyle, S. M. Fullerton, T. Ganiats, J. Hagenkord, S. Imhof, S. H. Rim, L. Ortmann, N. Aziz, W. D. Dotson, E. Matloff, K. Young, K. Kaphingst, A. Bradbury, J. Scott, C. Wang, A. Zauber, M. Levine, B. Korf, D. Leonard, C. Wicklund, G. Isham, and M. J. Khoury. 2018. A proposed approach for implementing genomics-based screening programs for healthy adults. *NAM Perspectives*. Washington, DC: National Academy of Medicine.

Nalls, M. A., C. Blauwendraat, C. L. Vallerga, K. Heilbron, S. Bandres-Ciga, D. Chang, M. Tan, D. A. Kia, A. J. Noyce, A. Xue, J. Bras, E. Young, R. von Coelln, J. Simón-Sánchez, C. Schulte, M. Sharma, L. Krohn, L. Pihlstrom, A. Siitonen, H. Iwaki, H. Leonard, F. Faghri, J. Raphael Gibbs, D. G. Hernandez, S. W. Scholz, J. A. Botia, M. Martinez, J.-C. Corvol, S. Lesage, J. Jankovic, L. M. Shulman, M. Sutherland, P. Tienari, K. Majamaa, M. Toft, O. A. Andreassen, T. Bangale, A. Brice, J. Yang, Z. Gan-Or, T. Gasser, P. Heutink, J. M. Shulman, N. Wood, D. A. Hinds, J. A. Hardy, H. R. Morris, J. Gratten, P. M. Visscher, R. R. Graham, and A. B. Singleton. 2019. Expanding Parkinson's disease genetics: Novel risk loci, genomic context, causal insights and heritable risk. *bioRxiv* 388165.

NASEM (National Academies of Sciences, Engineering, and Medicine). 2018. *Understanding disparities in access to genomic medicine: Proceedings of a workshop*. Washington, DC: The National Academies Press.

Nelson, S. C., J. H. Yu, J. K. Wagner, T. M. Harrell, C. D. Royal, and M. J. Bamshad. 2018. A content analysis of the views of genetics professionals on race, ancestry, and genetics. *AJOB Empirical Bioethics* 9(4):222–234.

Nelson, S. C., D. J. Bowen, and S. M. Fullerton. 2019. Third-party genetic interpretation tools: A mixed-methods study of consumer motivation and behavior. *American Journal of Human Genetics* 105(1):122–131.

Oliveri, S., F. Ferrari, A. Manfrinati, and G. Pravettoni. 2018. A systematic review of the psychological implications of genetic testing: A comparative analysis among cardiovascular, neurodegenerative and cancer diseases. *Frontiers in Genetics* 9:624.

Owusu Obeng, A., K. Fei, K. D. Levy, A. R. Elsey, T. I. Pollin, A. H. Ramirez, K. W. Weitzel, and C. R. Horowitz. 2018. Physician-reported benefits and barriers to clinical implementation of genomic medicine: A multi-site IGNITE-network survey. *Journal of Personalized Medicine* 8(3):24.

Personalized Medicine Coalition. 2018. *Public perspectives on personalized medicine: A survey of U.S. public opinion.* Washington, DC: Personalized Medicine Coalition.

Phillips, K. A., J. R. Trosman, and M. P. Douglas. 2019. Emergence of hybrid models of genetic testing beyond direct-to-consumer or traditional labs. *JAMA* 321(24):2403–2404.

Popejoy, A. B., and S. M. Fullerton. 2016. Genomics is failing on diversity. *Nature* 538(7624):161–164.

Popejoy, A. B., D. I. Ritter, K. Crooks, E. Currey, S. M. Fullerton, L. A. Hindorff, B. Koenig, E. M. Ramos, E. P. Sorokin, H. Wand, M. W. Wright, J. Zou, C. R. Gignoux, V. L. Bonham, S. E. Plon, and C. D. Bustamante. 2018. The clinical imperative for inclusivity: Race, ethnicity, and ancestry (REA) in genomics. *Human Mutation* 39(11):1713–1720.

Regalado, A. 2019. More than 26 million people have taken an at-home ancestry test. *MIT Technology Review*. https://www.technologyreview.com/s/612880/more-than-26-million-people-have-taken-an-at-home-ancestry-test (accessed January 23, 2020).

Roberts, J. S., M. C. Gornick, D. A. Carere, W. R. Uhlmann, M. T. Ruffin, and R. C. Green. 2017. Direct-to-consumer genetic testing: User motivations, decision making, and perceived utility of results. *Public Health Genomics* 20(1):36–45.

Rogers, E. 1962. *Diffusion of innovations, 3rd ed.* New York: The Free Press.

Roth, W. D., and B. Ivemark. 2018. Genetic options: The impact of genetic ancestry testing on consumers' racial and ethnic identities. *American Journal of Sociology* 124(1):150–184.

Royal, C. D., J. Novembre, S. M. Fullerton, D. B. Goldstein, J. C. Long, M. J. Bamshad, and A. G. Clark. 2010. Inferring genetic ancestry: Opportunities, challenges, and implications. *American Journal of Human Genetics* 86(5):661–673.

Salloum, R. G., T. J. George, N. Silver, M.-J. Markham, J. M. Hall, Y. Guo, J. Bian, and E. A. Shenkman. 2018. Rural–urban and racial-ethnic differences in awareness of direct-to-consumer genetic testing. *BMC Public Health* 18(1):277.

Shim, J. K., S. R. Alam, and B. E. Aouizerat. 2018. Knowing something versus feeling different: The effects and non-effects of genetic ancestry on racial identity. *New Genetics and Society* 37(1):44–66.

Sugrue, L. P., and R. S. Desikan. 2019. What are polygenic scores and why are they important? *JAMA* 321(18):1820–1821.

Sussner, K. M., H. S. Thompson, H. B. Valdimarsdottir, W. H. Redd, and L. Jandorf. 2009. Acculturation and familiarity with, attitudes towards and beliefs about genetic testing for cancer risk within Latinas in east Harlem, New York City. *Journal of Genetic Counseling* 18(1):60–71.

Tandy-Connor, S., J. Guiltinan, K. Krempely, H. LaDuca, P. Reineke, S. Gutierrez, P. Gray, and B. Tippin Davis. 2018. False-positive results released by direct-to-consumer genetic tests highlight the importance of clinical confirmation testing for appropriate patient care. *Genetics in Medicine* 20(12):1515–1521.

Ugalmugale, S. 2019. U.S. direct-to-consumer genetic testing market size by test type (carrier testing, predictive testing, ancestry & relationship testing, nutrigenomics testing), by technology (targeted analysis, single nucleotide polymorphism [SNP] chips, whole genome sequencing [WGS]), industry analysis report, application potential, competitive market share & forecast, 2019–2025. Global Market Insights, Inc. https://www.gminsights.com/industry-analysis/us-direct-to-consumer-genetic-testing-market (accessed January 9, 2020).

Vadaparampil, S. T., L. Wideroff, N. Breen, and E. Trapido. 2006. The impact of acculturation on awareness of genetic testing for increased cancer risk among Hispanics in the year 2000 National Health Interview survey. *Cancer Epidemiology, Biomarkers, and Prevention* 15(4):618–623.

Whitwell, S. C., C. G. Mathew, C. M. Lewis, A. Forbes, S. Watts, J. Sanderson, G. J. Hollands, A. T. Prevost, D. Armstrong, A. L. Kinmonth, S. Sutton, and T. M. Marteau. 2011. Trial protocol: Communicating DNA-based risk assessments for Crohn's disease: A randomised controlled trial assessing impact upon stopping smoking. *BMC Public Health* 11:44.

Wojcik, G. L., M. Graff, K. K. Nishimura, R. Tao, J. Haessler, C. R. Gignoux, H. M. Highland, Y. M. Patel, E. P. Sorokin, C. L. Avery, G. M. Belbin, S. A. Bien, I. Cheng, S. Cullina, C. J. Hodonsky, Y. Hu, L. M. Huckins, J. Jeff, A. E. Justice, J. M. Kocarnik, U. Lim, B. M. Lin, Y. Lu, S. C. Nelson, S.-S. L. Park, H. Poisner, M. H. Preuss, M. A. Richard, C. Schurmann, V. W. Setiawan, A. Sockell, K. Vahi, M. Verbanck, A. Vishnu, R. W. Walker, K. L. Young, N. Zubair, V. Acuña-Alonso, J. L. Ambite, K. C. Barnes, E. Boerwinkle, E. P. Bottinger, C. D. Bustamante, C. Caberto, S. Canizales-Quinteros, M. P. Conomos, E. Deelman, R. Do, K. Doheny, L. Fernández-Rhodes, M. Fornage, B. Hailu, G. Heiss, B. M. Henn, L. A. Hindorff, R. D. Jackson, C. A. Laurie, C. C. Laurie, Y. Li, D.-Y. Lin, A. Moreno-Estrada, G. Nadkarni, P. J. Norman, L. C. Pooler, A. P. Reiner, J. Romm, C. Sabatti, K. Sandoval, X. Sheng, E. A. Stahl, D. O. Stram, T. A. Thornton, C. L. Wassel, L. R. Wilkens, C. A. Winkler, S. Yoneyama, S. Buyske, C. A. Haiman, C. Kooperberg, L. Le Marchand, R. J. F. Loos, T. C. Matise, K. E. North, U. Peters, E. E. Kenny, and C. S. Carlson. 2019. Genetic analyses of diverse populations improves discovery for complex traits. *Nature* 570(7762):514–518.

Wolf, L. E., and L. M. Beskow. 2018. New and improved? 21st Century Cures Act revisions to certificates of confidentiality. *American Journal of Law and Medicine* 44(2–3):343–358.

Wright, C. F., and S. Gregory-Jones. 2010. Size of the direct-to-consumer genomic testing market. *Genetics in Medicine* 12(9):594.

Appendix A

Workshop Agenda

Exploring the Current Landscape of Consumer Genomics—
A Workshop

October 29, 2019

Keck Building of the National Academies
500 Fifth Street, NW
Room 100
Washington, DC 20001

8:30 a.m. **Opening Remarks**

GEOFFREY GINSBURG, *Roundtable Co-Chair*
Director, Duke Center for Applied Genomics & Precision Medicine
Professor, Medicine, Pathology, and Biomedical Engineering
Duke University Medical Center

MICHELLE PENNY, *Roundtable Co-Chair*
Head of Translational Genome Sciences
Biogen

8:35 a.m. **Charge to Workshop Speakers and Participants**

GREG FEERO, *Workshop Co-Chair*
Professor, Department of Community and Family Medicine
Geisel School of Medicine
Faculty, Maine Dartmouth Family Medical Residency Program
Associate Editor, *Journal of the American Medical Association*

CATHY WICKLUND, *Workshop Co-Chair*
Director, Graduate Program in Genetic Counseling
Past President, National Society of Genetic Counselors
Associate Professor, Feinberg School of Medicine, Center for Genetic Medicine
Northwestern University

8:50 a.m. **Opening Keynote**

ROBERT NUSSBAUM
Chief Medical Officer
Invitae

9:10 a.m. **Clarifying Questions from Workshop Participants**

SESSION I: UNDERSTANDING CONSUMER GENOMICS UTILIZATION

Session Objectives:

- Explore how consumers are engaging (or not engaging) with direct-to-consumer and consumer-driven genomics services and whether there are lessons that can be learned about overall health engagement
- Learn how patients and providers are using genomic data procured through consumer genomics applications along with health data from other sources to inform overall health care decision making

Session Moderator: Tina Hesman Saey, Science News

9:15 a.m. **Consumer Genomics Engagement and Outlook**

CINNAMON BLOSS
Associate Professor
Departments of Psychiatry and Family Medicine and Public Health
University of California, San Diego

9:30 a.m. **Consumer Perspectives**

Sara Altschule
Freelance Writer
Bustle Magazine

Dorothy Pomerantz
Managing Editor
FitchInk

10:00 a.m. **Panel Discussion with Speakers and Workshop Participants**

10:30 a.m. **Break**

SESSION II: EXPLORING THE ROLE OF DIVERSITY AND HEALTH DISPARITIES IN CONSUMER GENOMICS

Session Objectives:

- Discuss the lack of diversity in current genomics databases and biorepositories and how this may affect health disparities
- Explore how consumer genomics is (or is not) reaching diverse populations (e.g., racial, ethnic, geographic, socioeconomic) and the implications for health disparities

Session Moderator: Jacquelyn Taylor, New York University

10:45 a.m. Joyce Tung
Vice President, Research
23andMe

11:00 a.m. Malia Fullerton
Professor of Bioethics and Humanities
University of Washington School of Medicine

11:15 a.m. Shawneequa Callier
Associate Professor of Clinical Research and Leadership
The George Washington University

11:30 a.m. Sadie Hutson
Director, Cancer Genetics Program
Pikeville Medical Center
Assistant Dean, Graduate Programs
University of Tennessee, Knoxville

11:45 a.m. **Panel Discussion with Speakers and Workshop Participants**

12:30 p.m. **Working Lunch**

SESSION III: INTEGRATION WITHIN SCIENTIFIC AND MEDICAL COMMUNITIES

Session Objectives:

- Discuss factors that may affect how consumer genomics data are integrated with clinical care
- Examine the challenges of and opportunities for using consumer genomics for research
- Explore emerging cross-sector collaborations and potential lessons that can be learned

Session Moderator: Bruce Blumberg, Kaiser Permanente School of Medicine

1:30 p.m. ANDREW SINGLETON
Senior Investigator
Laboratory of Neurogenetics
National Institute on Aging

1:45 p.m. SIOBHAN DOLAN
Professor and Vice Chair for Research
Department of Obstetrics and Gynecology and Women's Health
Albert Einstein College of Medicine

2:00 p.m. DANIELLE BONADIES
Director of Genetics
My Gene Counsel

2:15 p.m. MATTHEW FERBER
Associate Professor of Laboratory Medicine and Pathology
Consultant, Division of Laboratory Genetics and Genomics, Department of Laboratory Medicine and Pathology
Mayo Clinic

2:30 p.m. **Panel Discussion with Speakers and Workshop Participants**

3:00 p.m. **Break**

SESSION IV: REGULATORY AND HEALTH POLICY ISSUES

Session Objectives:

- Address data sharing, privacy, and security issues in the context of consumer genomics testing
- Explore the landscape of emerging regulatory issues in consumer genomics

Session Moderator: Victoria M. Pratt, Association for Molecular Pathology

3:15 p.m. AMY MCGUIRE
Leon Jaworski Professor Biomedical Ethics
Director, Center for Medical Ethics and Health Policy
Baylor College of Medicine

3:30 p.m. GAIL JAVITT
Member, Health Care and Life Sciences Practice
Epstein Becker Green

3:45 p.m. JORDAN LASER
Senior Director
Cytogenetics and Molecular Pathology of Pathology and Laboratory Medicine
Long Island Jewish Medical Center

4:00 p.m. **Panel Discussion with Speakers and Workshop Participants**

SESSION V: HOW CAN CONSUMER GENOMICS BE BETTER INTEGRATED TO IMPROVE HEALTH?

Session Objectives:

- What is the role of consumer genomics in the health care system in the next 5 years? 10 years?
  - What is viewed as actionable information by a health system?
- Are health systems, consumers, and providers prepared for downstream challenges? If not, are there opportunities for ensuring that consumer genomics is more effective in clinical care?
- How can we make consumer genomics the best it can be for consumers and systems?
  - What needs to be better understood about low-cost consumer genomics and the implications for access and health disparities?

Session Moderator: Huntington Willard, Geisinger National Precision Health

4:30 p.m. **Reflections on the Day and Next Steps**

Danielle Bonadies
Shawneequa Callier
Siobhan Dolan
Robert Nussbaum
Dorothy Pomerantz

Additional Discussant:

Timothy Stenzel
Director, Office of In Vitro Diagnostics and Radiological Health
Office of Product Evaluation and Quality
Center for Devices and Radiological Health
Food and Drug Administration

5:00 p.m. **Final Discussion with Workshop Participants**

5:20 p.m. **Final Remarks from Workshop Co-Chairs**

Greg Feero, *Workshop Co-Chair*
Professor, Department of Community and Family Medicine
Geisel School of Medicine
Faculty, Maine Dartmouth Family Medical Residency Program
Associate Editor, *Journal of the American Medical Association*

Cathy Wicklund, Workshop Co-Chair
Director, Graduate Program in Genetic Counseling
Past President, National Society of Genetic Counselors
Associate Professor, Feinberg School of Medicine, Center for Genetic Medicine
Northwestern University

5:35 p.m. **Adjourn**
Networking Reception

Appendix B

Speaker Biographical Sketches

Sara Altschule, a *BRCA 2* carrier, is an advocate for women's health and empowerment. She has documented her experience of discovering her *BRCA* mutation to undergoing a preventive double mastectomy with reconstruction for various publications (*Bustle*, *SELF*, *Refinery29*, and more).

Cinnamon Bloss, Ph.D., is an associate professor in the Department of Family Medicine and Public Health, Division of Health Policy at the University of California, San Diego. Dr. Bloss has secondary appointments in the Departments of Psychiatry and Medicine (Division of Biomedical Informatics) and is a licensed clinical psychologist. The primary focus of Dr. Bloss's work is interdisciplinary research on the individual and societal impacts of emerging biomedical technologies. With a background in clinical psychology, statistical genetics, and biomedical ethics, she has conducted large-scale projects in areas such as direct-to-consumer genomics, genome sequencing in diagnostic odyssey cases, privacy and big data, and genome editing. Dr. Bloss has been the principal investigator or a co-investigator on more than 15 federal grants, has published more than 80 papers, and mentored more than 40 students.

Danielle Bonadies, M.S., C.G.C., is the director of the genetics division at My Gene Counsel, a digital health company that links current, updating, evidence-based information to genetic test results. Ms. Bonadies practiced as a clinical genetic counselor at the Yale School of Medicine for a decade, where she was the assistant director of the Cancer Genetic Counseling Program. She designed and ran several interactive, online patient education and communication sites and was involved in the cancer genetics education of thousands of patients, clinicians, and students. Ms. Bonadies has co-authored multiple book chapters and articles on genetic counseling and testing and was involved in the collection, documentation, and publication of several key articles about the high rate of result misinterpretation among clinicians ordering genetic testing. At My Gene Counsel, Ms. Bonadies oversees the development of digital genetic counseling tools and takes an active role in technology development.

Shawneequa Callier, J.D., M.A., is an associate professor in the Department of Clinical Research and Leadership at The George Washington University School of Medicine and Health Sciences (SMHS). Dr. Callier teaches courses in bioethics and health care law in a variety of programs at SMHS. She is also a professorial lecturer in law at The George Washington University Law School and a special volunteer at the Center for Research on Genomics and Global Health, National Human Genome Research Institute, National Institutes of Health. Dr. Callier's research focuses on issues at the intersection of bioethics, law, genomics, and emerging technologies.

Siobhan M. Dolan, M.D., M.P.H., is a professor and the vice chair for research in the Department of Obstetrics and Gynecology and Women's Health at the Albert Einstein College of Medicine and the Montefiore Medical Center in the Bronx. Board-certified in both obstetrics/gynecology and clinical genetics, she maintains her clinical practice in the Division of Reproductive and Medical Genetics at Montefiore where she works to improve the health of mothers and children by preventing birth defects, preterm birth, and infant mortality.

Matthew Ferber, Ph.D., is an assistant professor and a consultant in the Department of Laboratory Medicine and Pathology at the Mayo Clinic, where he serves as a co-director for the Genomics Laboratory. He was the founder and the director of the Clinical Genome Sequencing Laboratory at Mayo from 2012 to 2018. He has worked very closely with Mayo Clinic's Center for Individualized Medicine over the years, serving as a founding member of the Clinomics program, which created the Individualized Medicine Clinic and Mayo's Diagnostic Odyssey Services. In October 2018, under the leadership of Dr. Ferber, Mayo's consumer genomic testing product, Mayo Clinic GeneGuide™, was launched.

Stephanie Malia Fullerton, D.Phil., is a professor of bioethics and humanities at the University of Washington (UW) School of Medicine. She is also an adjunct professor in the UW departments of epidemiology, genome sciences, and medicine (medical genetics) as well as an affiliate investigator with the

Public Health Sciences division of the Fred Hutchinson Cancer Research Center. She received a Ph.D. in human population genetics from the University of Oxford and later re-trained in ethical, legal, and social implications (ELSI) research with a fellowship from the National Human Genome Research Institute at the National Institutes of Health. Dr. Fullerton's work focuses on the ethical and social implications of genomic research and its equitable and safe translation for clinical and public health benefit. She serves as the ELSI lead for the Clinical Sequencing Evidence-Generating Research (CSER2) Consortium coordinating center, co-chairs the TOPMed Consortium ELSI Committee, and chairs the bioethics advisory board of the Kaiser Permanente Research Bank. She contributes to a range of empirical projects focused on clinical genomics translation and precision medicine approaches to the treatment and prevention of cancer and kidney disease in diverse patient populations.

Sadie Hutson, Ph.D., R.N., WHNP-BC, FAANP, is currently a professor and an assistant dean of graduate programs at the University of Tennessee College of Nursing. She earned a Ph.D. in nursing and an M.S.N. as a women's health nurse practitioner from the University of Pennsylvania in Philadelphia. Dr. Hutson additionally received a B.S.N. from the University of Wisconsin–Madison and a certificate in clinical genetics from Georgetown University. Her areas of scientific interest include studying the consequences of living with chronic illness in rural and underserved areas, specifically Appalachia. Dr. Hutson practices clinically as the director of the cancer genetics program at the Leonard Lawson Cancer Center at the Pikeville Medical Center in eastern Kentucky.

Gail H. Javitt, J.D., M.P.H., is a member of the firm in the health care and life sciences practice in the Washington, DC, office of Epstein Becker Green. Ms. Javitt provides strategic Food and Drug Administration (FDA) regulatory advice for leading medical device, diagnostics, pharmaceutical, biological products, human cellular, and tissue-based products (HCT/Ps) and dietary supplement companies throughout the product life cycle, and she has successfully resolved disputes at both the pre- and postmarket stage. She also has significant experience advising clinical laboratories on FDA and the Clinical Laboratory Improvement Amendments requirements for laboratory-developed tests. Ms. Javitt's experience prior to joining Epstein Becker Green included serving as counsel in a major Washington, DC, FDA regulatory practice and as a law and policy director at the Genetics and Public Policy Center, part of Johns Hopkins University. At the center, she was responsible for developing policy options to guide the development and use of reproductive and other genetic technologies. In addition, Ms. Javitt has published and spoken widely on issues at the intersection of law and science, including FDA regulation of genetic testing, precision medicine, and next-generation sequencing. Her academic experience has included serving as a faculty member at the Berman Institute of Bioethics at Johns Hopkins University and as an adjunct professor at the Georgetown University Law Center, American University's Washington College of Law, and the University of Maryland School of Law. She was previously a Greenwall Fellow in Bioethics and Health Policy, a collaborative effort between Johns Hopkins University and Georgetown University.

Jordan Laser, M.D., is a board-certified anatomic, clinical, and molecular genetic pathologist. Currently employed at Northwell Health System in New York, Dr. Laser serves the Department of Pathology and Laboratory Medicine in the following roles: medical director, Long Island Jewish Medical Center pathology and laboratory medicine; associate medical director, Core Laboratories; senior director, Division of Cytogenetics and Molecular Pathology; and director, Division of Near Patient Testing. Dr. Laser is active in key pathology professional societies such as the Association for Molecular Pathology, where he chairs the Professional Relations Committee, and the College of American Pathologists, where he is the vice chair of the Personalized Healthcare Committee. His expertise includes molecular and genomic medicine, laboratory management, health care finance, and standards and regulations.

Amy McGuire, J.D., Ph.D., is the Leon Jaworski Professor of Biomedical Ethics and the director of the Center for Medical Ethics and Health Policy at the Baylor College of Medicine. She researches ethical and policy issues in human genetics, with a particular focus on genomic research and the clinical integration of emerging technologies. Currently, she is studying issues related to genomic data sharing, the policy implications of emerging business models for next-generation sequencing, and ethical and policy issues arising in the clinical integration of genomic technologies. Her research is funded by the National Human Genome Research Institute, the National Cancer Institute, and the National Institute of Child Health and Human Development at the National Institutes of Health, and she is a member of the advisory committee for the Greenwall Faculty Scholars Program in Bioethics.

Robert Nussbaum, M.D., is the chief medical officer of Invitae, a genetic information and diagnostic company. He is board certified in internal medicine, clinical genetics, and clinical molecular genetics and is a fellow of the American College of Physicians and the American College of Medical Genetics and Genomics. From 2006 to 2015 he was the Holly Smith Professor of Medicine at the University of California, San Francisco (UCSF), and the chief of the Division of Genomic Medicine and Medical Director of both the cancer risk program and the UCSF program in cardiovascular genetics. He previously served in the Division of Intramural Research of the National Human Genome Research Institute of the National Institutes of Health and was a professor of human genetics, pediatrics, and medicine at the University of Pennsylvania and an associate investigator of the Howard Hughes Medical Institute. He received an M.D. in 1975 from the Harvard–Massachusetts Institute of Technology joint program in health science and technology, internal medicine training at Barnes Hospital/Washington University (1975–1978), and genetics training at the Baylor College of Medicine (1978–1981). He is the co-author of more than 230 peer-reviewed publications in basic and applied human genetics as well as numerous commentaries, editorials, and textbook chapters. He was elected to the National Academy of Medicine in 2004 and to the American Academy of Arts & Sciences in 2015. Dr. Nussbaum served as a member of the board of directors and as the president of the American Society of Human Genetics, was on the board of directors of the American Board of Medical Genetics and Genomics, and was a founding fellow on the board of directors of the American College of Medical Genetics and Genomics. Dr. Nussbaum was awarded the Klaus Joachim Zülch-Prize for Neurological Research, the Jay Van Andel Award for Outstanding Achievement in Parkinson's Disease Research, and the Calne Lectureship from Parkinson Canada for his work on hereditary Parkinson disease. He is co-author with Drs. Roderick M. McInnes and Huntington F. Willard of three editions of the popular textbook of human genetics, *Thompson and Thompson's Genetics in Medicine*. With his two co-authors, he received the 2015 Award for Excellence in Human Genetics Education from the American Society of Human Genetics. He has received numerous other awards for research, service, and education from the University of Pennsylvania, the National Institutes of Health, UCSF, and the Lowe Syndrome Association.

Dorothy Pomerantz is a writer, editor, and strategist. In 2018 she did an at-home genetics test on a whim and received terrible health news. She is sharing her story in the hope of helping people who will find themselves in the same situation.

Andrew Singleton, Ph.D., received his B.Sc. from the University of Sunderland, United Kingdom, and his Ph.D. from the University of Newcastle upon Tyne, United Kingdom. His research initially focused on the genetic determinants of dementia, in particular Alzheimer's disease and dementia with Lewy bodies. His postdoctoral studies were spent at the Mayo Clinic in Jacksonville, Florida. Dr. Singleton moved to the National Institute on Aging (NIA) at the National Institutes of Health (NIH) in Bethesda, Maryland, in

2001 and became a principal investigator leading the Molecular Genetics Unit in 2002. In 2007 Dr. Singleton became a tenured senior investigator at NIA, in 2008 he became the chief of the Laboratory of Neurogenetics, and in 2016 he was named an NIH distinguished investigator. Dr. Singleton has published more than 550 articles on a wide variety of topics. His laboratory comprises approximately 50 staff, including 5 principal investigators and 3 group leaders. His laboratory works on the genetic basis of neurological disorders including Parkinson's disease, Alzheimer's disease, dystonia, ataxia, dementia with Lewy bodies, and amyotrophic lateral sclerosis. The goal of this research is to identify genetic variability that causes or contributes to disease and to use this knowledge to understand the molecular processes underlying disease. Most recently his work has expanded to the use of multimodal data in predicting disease. Dr. Singleton currently serves on the scientific advisory board of The Michael J. Fox Foundation for Parkinson's Research and the Lewy Body Dementia Association; he is a member of the editorial boards of *Neurodegenerative Diseases*, *Neurobiology of Disease* (associate editor, genetics), *Neurogenetics*, *Movement Disorders*, *Brain* (associate editor, genetics), *Lancet Neurology*, the *Journal of Parkinson's Disease*, *NPJ Parkinson's Disease* (associate editor), and the *Journal of Huntington's Disease*. Dr. Singleton was awarded the Boehringer Mannheim Research Award in 2005, the NIH Director's Award in 2008 and again in 2016, and the Annemarie Opprecht Award for Parkinson's disease research in 2008. In 2012 Dr. Singleton became the first person to win the Jay van Andel Award for Outstanding Achievement in Parkinson's Disease Research. In 2017 Dr. Singleton was awarded the American Academy of Neurology Movement Disorders Award and an honorary doctorate from his alma mater, the University of Sunderland.

Timothy Stenzel, M.D., Ph.D., joined the Food and Drug Administration (FDA) in July 2018 and has an extensive background, spanning more than 20 years, in executive leadership, innovation, companion diagnostics, research and development, FDA regulations, and clinical laboratory operations. He received his M.D. and Ph.D. in microbiology and immunology, focusing on the molecular biology of DNA replication, from Duke University after graduating with honors in chemistry from Grinnell College. In his last position, from 2014 to 2018, Dr. Stenzel served as the chief operating officer at Invivoscribe, focusing on companion diagnostics and next-generation sequencing/massively parallel sequencing in oncology. During his career he has played important roles in the development and launch of more than 30 in vitro diagnostic products, as well as numerous unique laboratory-developed test services, including the FDA-approved companion diagnostic for Novartis's drug Rydapt and the world's first clinical microRNA assay (for pancreatic cancer detection). Other experience includes serving as the chief scientific officer and the founder of the Molecular Diagnostics franchise at Quidel, the chief medical officer and the vice president of research and development at Asuragen, and the senior director for medical, regulatory, and clinical affairs at Abbott Molecular. Dr. Stenzel served as a board director at the American College of Medical Genetics and Genomics (ACMG) Foundation for Genetic and Genomic Medicine from 2008 to 2013. He has served on the ACMG/College of American Pathologists (CAP) Biochemical and Molecular Genetics Resource Committee from 1996 to 2005, the Association for Molecular Pathology (AMP) finance committee from 2012 to 2018, the AMP strategic planning committee from 2007 to 2009, as the AMP chair-elect and chair of the Solid Tumor Division from 2003 to 2004, the CAP molecular oncology committee from 2013 to 2018, and as a member of the CAP house of delegates from 2011 to 2017. As the Office of In Vitro Diagnostics and Radiological Health (OIR) director at FDA, Dr. Stenzel will advise center leadership on all regulatory (premarket and postmarket) in vitro diagnostic, radiological medical device, and radiation-emitting product issues that have an impact on center- and agency-level decisions, policy development, nationwide program execution and short- and long-range program goals and objectives as well as provide executive leadership and scientific direction to the OIR staff.

Joyce Tung, Ph.D., joined 23andMe in 2007 and manages the 23andMe research team, which is responsible for consumer health and ancestry research and development, academic and industry collaborations, computational analyses for therapeutics, and new research methods and tools development. While a postdoctoral fellow at Stanford University, Dr. Tung studied the genetics of mouse and human pigmentation. She graduated from Stanford with honors and distinction with a B.S. in biological sciences and a minor in computer science, and she earned her Ph.D. in genetics from the University of California, San Francisco, where she was a National Science Foundation graduate research fellow.

Appendix C

Statement of Task

Consumer genomics, encompassing both direct-to-consumer (DTC) applications (i.e., genetic testing that is accessed by a consumer directly from a commercial company apart from a health care provider) and consumer-driven genetic testing (i.e., genetic testing ordered by a health care provider in response to an informed patient request), has evolved considerably over the past decade, moving from more personal utility–focused applications outside of traditional health care to interfacing with clinical care in non-traditional ways. As consumer genomics has increasingly intersected with clinical applications, discussions have arisen around the need to demonstrate clinical and analytical validity and clinical utility due to the potential for misinterpretation by consumers. Clinical readiness and interest for this information have presented educational and training challenges for providers. At the same time, consumer genomics has emerged as a potentially innovative mechanism for thinking about health literacy and engaging participants in their health and health care.

An ad hoc planning committee will plan and conduct a 1-day public workshop to explore the current landscape of consumer genomics and implications for how genetic test information is used or may be used in research and clinical care. Discussions may include topics such as diversity of participant populations, impact on health literacy and engagement, knowledge gaps related to use in clinical care, and data privacy/security concerns. A broad array of stakeholders may take part in the workshop, including genomics and consumer genomics experts, epidemiologists, health disparities researchers, clinicians, users of consumer genomics research applications (e.g., consumers, patients), patient advocacy groups, payers, bioethicists, regulators, and policy makers. The planning committee will develop the workshop agenda, select and invite speakers and discussants, and may moderate the discussions. A proceedings of the presentations and discussions at the workshop will be prepared by a designated rapporteur in accordance with institutional guidelines.

Appendix D

Registered Attendees

Lori Achman
Government Accountability Office

Joseph Alper
Science Writer

Joyce Altschule
Individual

Sara Altschule
Consumer

Maria Arif
Howard University

Naomi Aronson
Blue Cross and Blue Shield Association

Cynthia Bens
Personalized Medicine Coalition

Adam Berger
National Institutes of Health

Karina Bienfait
Merck and Co., Inc.

Barbara Biesecker
RTI International

Cinnamon Bloss
University of California, San Diego

Bruce Blumberg
Kaiser Permanente School of Medicine

Danielle Bonadies
My Gene Counsel

Vence Bonham
National Human Genome Research Institute

Natasha Bonhomme
Genetic Alliance

Megan Anderson Brooks
Innovation Policy Solutions

Shawneequa Callier
The George Washington University

Ariadne Campble
The Washington Center

Elaine Collier
National Center for Advancing Translational Sciences

Kayla Cooper
National Institutes of Health

Thao Dinh
Johns Hopkins University

Andrea Jackson Dipina
National Institutes of Health

Michael Dobias
The Pew Charitable Trusts

Siobhan Dolan
Albert Einstein College of Medicine/Montefiore Medical Center

Emily Edelman
The Jackson Laboratory

Christin Engelhardt
American Cancer Society Cancer Action Network

Grace-Ann Fasaye
National Cancer Institute

W. Gregory Feero
Journal of the American Medical Association

Matthew Ferber
Mayo Clinic

Tempora Fisher
National Institutes of Health

Mark Fleury
American Cancer Society Cancer Action Network

Megan Frone
National Cancer Institute

Stephanie Malia Fullerton
University of Washington

Ann Geiger
National Cancer Institute

Kenneth Getz
Tufts University School of Medicine

Elena Ghanaim
National Human Genome Research Institute

Geoffrey Ginsburg
Duke University

Aaron Goldenberg
Case Western Reserve University School of Medicine

Eve Granatosky
American Society of Human Genetics

Nasreen Haque
New York Medical College

Alaina Harris
Health Resources and Services Administration

Rebecca Helgesen
Penn Medicine

Kathy Helzlsouer
National Cancer Institute

Ross Henderson
CAREM, LLC

Marvin Higgins
Yoga for Peace, Joy and Love

Brittany Hollister
National Human Genome Research Institute

Gillian Hooker
National Society of Genetic Counselors

Alejandra Hurtado
Georgetown University

Sadie Hutson
University of Tennessee, Knoxville

Mira Irons
American Medical Association

Praduman Jain
Vibrent Health

Gail Javitt
Epstein Becker Green

Richard Jordan
Blue Community Consortium

Cristina Kapustij
National Human Genome Research Institute

Robert Karp
National Institute of Diabetes and Digestive and Kidney Diseases

Manjula Kasoji
Booz Allen Hamilton

Samata Katta
American Society of Human Genetics/National Human Genome Research Institute

Soohyun Kim
Health Resources and Services Administration

William Klein
National Cancer Institute/National Institutes of Health

Danuta Krotoski
National Institute of Child Health and Human Development

Kailey Lamb
The George Washington University Medical Faculty Associates

Katherine Lamberson
Genetic Alliance

Kristofor Langlais
National Institutes of Health

Jordan Laser
Northwell Health

Gabriela Lavezzari
GlaxoSmithKline

Alexandra Lebensohn
National Institutes of Health

Jennifer Leib
Innovation Policy Solutions

Charles Macri
The George Washington University

Jean-Claude Marshall
Pfizer Inc.

Michelle McClure
American College of Medical Genetics and Genomics

Sean McConnell
American Medical Association

Amy McGuire
Baylor College of Medicine Center for Medical Ethics and Health Policy

George Mensah
National Heart, Lung, and Blood Institute

Wynn Meyer
National Institutes of Health

Mona Miller
American Society of Human Genetics

Allison Miner
Kaiser Permanente

Timothy Morck
Spectrum Nutrition, LLC

Christiane Morecock
The George Washington University Medical Faculty Associates

Maximilian Muenke
American College of Medical Genetics and Genomics

Gregory Nacarelli
Johns Hopkins University

Phillip Nichols
Gwood llc

Robert Nussbaum
Invitae

Kristina Obom
Johns Hopkins University

Jeanne O'Brien
Shady Grove Fertility

Natasha Pacheco
Inova Translational Medicine Institute

Cindy Paredes
Corazón Latino

Michelle Penny
Biogen

Valentina Petkov
National Cancer Institute

Anna Pettersson
Pfizer Inc.

María Pfund
Congressional Hispanic Caucus Institute

Dorothy Pomerantz
FitchInk

Victoria Pratt
Association for Molecular Pathology

Daryl Pritchard
Personalized Medicine Coalition

Nalini Raghavachari
National Institute on Aging

Pratima Rayavarapu
Johns Hopkins University

Jessica Reusch
National Institutes of Health

Catharine Riley
Health Resources and Services Administration

Laura Lyman Rodriguez
Geisinger National Precision Health

Ella Saccon
National Cancer Institute

Tina Saey
Science News

Meredith Safford
Johns Hopkins University

Faswilla Sampson
Personalized Medicine Coalition

Kunal Sanghavi
The Jackson Laboratory

V. Schneider
National Aeronautics and Space Administration

Derek Scholes
American Society of Human Genetics

Emma Schopp
National Human Genome Research Institute

Melissa Schweitzer
Human Longevity, Inc.

Joan Scott
Health Resources and Services Administration

Geetha Senthil
National Institute of Mental Health

Sam Shekar
Consultant

Nonniekaye Shelburne
National Cancer Institute

Niki Sidiropoulos
The University of Vermont Health Network Medical Group

Hilary Silver
The George Washington University

Andrew Singleton
National Institute on Aging

Emily Smith
CBR, a California Cryobank Life Sciences Company

Kayla Smith
Personalized Medicine Coalition

Gabriel Soto
IADF

Nina Sperber
Duke University

Angela Starkweather
University of Connecticut

Timothy Stenzel
Food and Drug Administration

Coco Stewart
National Human Genome Research Institute

Ryan Taft
Illumina, Inc.

Jacquelyn Taylor
New York University College of Nursing and School of Medicine

Sharon Terry
Genetic Alliance

Parmi Shailesh Thakker
Johns Hopkins University

Naiju Thomas
Johns Hopkins University

Austin Thompson
Technology and Media Initiative

Darla Thompson
Robert Wood Johnson Foundation Health Policy Research Scholars/The George Washington University

Linda Thompson
Howard University

Lois Tully
National Institute of Nursing Research

Joyce Tung
23andMe

Camila Valencia
Inter-American Development Bank

Amanda Vernon
American Academy of Arts & Sciences

Vivian Ota Wang
National Cancer Institute

Michael Watson
American College of Medical Genetics and Genomics

Karen Weck
University of North Carolina School of Medicine

Catherine Wicklund
Northwestern University

Huntington Willard
Geisinger National Precision Health

Beth Wilmot
National Institute on Aging

Anier Landon Woodyard
Innovatio Et Cetera Corporation

Sarah Wordsworth
University of Oxford

Yining Xie
GS

Alicia Zhou
Color Genomics